Dr Franz Wagner

Acupressure

Healing techniques using gentle pressure and self-massage

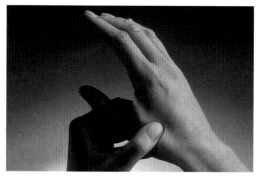

Effective self-help to:

- relieve pain

- promote relaxation

- stimulate the body's energy

TIME-LIFE BOOKS, AMSTERDAM

Contents

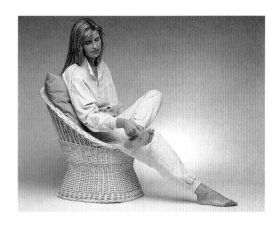

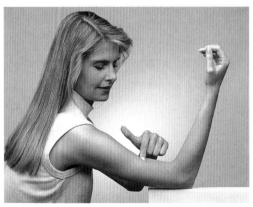

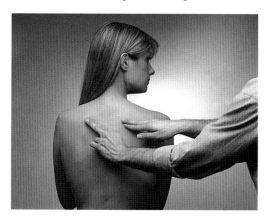

For Annaliese and Gaston – the fount of my strength.

Important

The views expressed by the authors of the HEALTH CARE TODAY
series may differ at times from generally recognized orthodox
medicine. All readers must decide for themselves whether, and to
what extent, they wish to follow the natural healing methods in
this book. If you want to use acupressure techniques in support of
another medical therapy, please make sure you consult your
doctor first.

All the instructions given in this book have been proven to
work in practice. However, every person reacts differently to
treatment, and success depends to an extent on the skill and care
with which the treatment is carried out. Self-treatment demands a
high degree of responsibility on the part of the individual. Before
commencing any treatment, please make sure you have read and
understood the instructions, and always follow the advice on
preparation and the rules of treatment (see pages 33-37 and 40).

Foreword

Acupressure has been used in China for thousands of years and is one of the oldest and most proven natural healing methods. As with other natural healing methods that have come from the East, acupressure does not deal with illness or physical problems in isolation. A person is seen as a single unit comprising body, soul and spirit. All physical disorders are considered within this context and treatment is always directed at the whole body-soul-spirit unit. Therefore local symptoms are considered to be an expression of the condition of the body as a whole and acupuncture is used to cure both the symptom and the underlying reason for the illness.

Proven for thousands of years

Acupressure uses the same pressure points as acupuncture, but instead of needles, acupressure uses the gentle but firm pressure of the hands and feet.

Acupuncture is also used to balance the body and to maintain good health. It can reduce tension, increase circulation and enable the body to relax deeply. By relieving stress and balancing the forces within the body, acupuncture can strengthen our resistance to disease and help promote health.

Striving for balance

Health is the constant battle of the forces within us for balance. If these forces are blocked by anything, we find ourselves in an unbalanced condition that leads to bodily disorders – then we become ill.

Setting free blocked energy   With acupressure we can influence the flow of our energy, we can redirect misguided energy via certain nerve centres and we can set free blocked energy. Where the cause of any disorder is due to an imbalance of the forces within us, we can use acupressure to treat the illness.

Help from our own vitality

With acupressure, which is also called pressure point massage, we have a natural healing method at our disposal. Acupressure enables us to look after our own health by using the forces within us – to help ourselves from within. Acupressure is a natural, original, very reliable, effective and nearly pain-free method of treatment.

Everyone can use acupressure: the success of treatment does not rely on specific medical knowledge and there is no fear of any damaging side-effects. The healing method can be used without the need for any technical appliances and in nearly any situation with very little effort. Once you know the acupressure points and the effects they will have, bodily disorders can quickly be eliminated by massaging these points.   **Acupressure for everyone**

With acupressure your own well-being is actually "in your hands", so that you can look after your own health. Once you have learnt where the important pressure points are you will never miss these points again. Everyone who suffers from complaints like **Reliable, without any side-effects**   headaches, back pains, migraine, sore throats or colds would probably like to be able to lay their hands on a quick, problem-free solution – especially one that was also free of side-effects. Acupressure can be this solution – for all of us.

A prerequisite for the success of a treatment with acupressure is the willingness to be responsible for your own health. This natural method of treatment is based on thousands of years of experience. Through these experiences we learn that self-treatment helps us to recognise the important signals that our bodies give us. It is quite usual for people to develop a better relationship with their bodies through experiences of self-treatment. Natural healers say that healing only starts when the person being treated takes up contact with their own body.

Recognising the signals

Please Note:

Acupressure can never replace any prescribed medical treatment thought necessary: it can however be a useful supplement to other forms of therapy as a natural healing method. If you are already undergoing treatment and also want to treat your complaints with acupressure, you should always consult your doctor first.

All forms of natural self-treatment require initiative and responsibility, as well as patience and perseverance when putting the treatment into practice. If you follow the advice and instructions in this book, you will learn how to use acupressure to help you heal everyday complaints and pains, naturally.

Patience is important

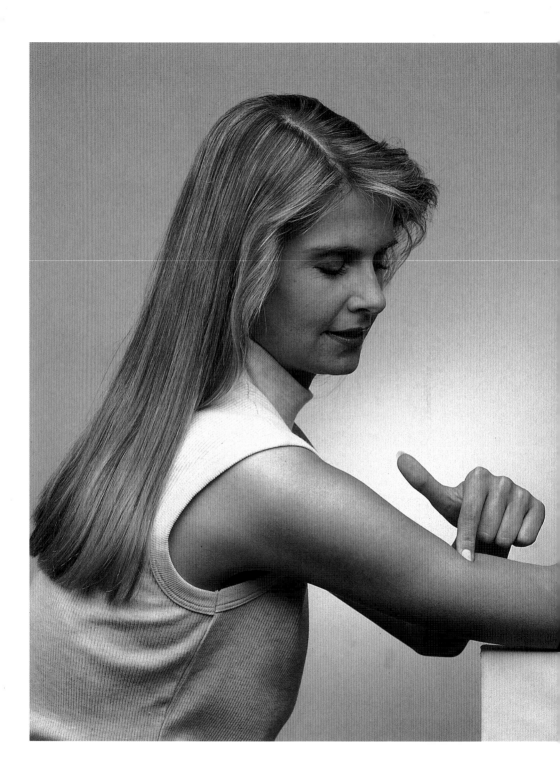

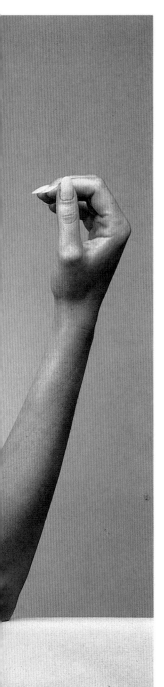

A holistic healing method

All natural healing methods are based on the holistic principle that a person is a "whole" being made up of body, mind and spirit. In diagnosing and treating illness it is just as important to consider the condition of the mind as it is to examine the body. Conventional western medicine tends to regard the ill body as a machine in need of repair which can be restored to working order through the application of external influences. In contrast, acupressure works with the body to stimulate the flow of a person's natural energy and strengthen their own self-healing forces. This is the basic premise by which natural healing methods differentiate themselves from Western orthodox medicine.

What does holistic mean?

When successful treatments confound accepted scientific wisdom and surprise the human imagination, it is often because our understanding of how the human body works is mistaken or incomplete. The capacity of the human body to heal and rejuvenate itself is truly amazing, and whenever we express wonder at an example of healing we are simply demonstrating our failure to appreciate this potential.

Our underestimation of the body's healing ability is largely due to the fact that we have forgotten how the body works and reacts. The human body expresses itself quite clearly and fluently – but in the modern world we have forgotten how to listen to it. We need to learn to consider the human body in a holistic light once more, and in so doing adopt a new perception of health and illness.

Inner balance of forces

A "new" understanding of health

In the East, health is viewed as a question of balance, and in fact this perception is not so new to the West. The ancient Greek physician Hippocrates – who lived from 460-377 BC and framed medicine's famous Hippocratic Oath – regarded health as a balance of forces. It followed that illness was the result of a malfunction of this balance, while healing was a process of re-establishing the body's balance.

Some two millennia later, the famous Swiss physician Paracelsus (1493-1541) described our primary healing power as the "inner-being doctor", or the "doctor within ourselves". The healing process depended on setting free forces inside the body which can restore its natural balance and make it function properly again. These healing forces are often hidden, submerged or misguided. Not only have we forgotten how to mobilise them, often we are actually working against them. The holistic healing sciences aim to

The "inner-being doctor"

harness the body's healing forces and support our natural defence mechanisms instead of suppressing them. For example, rather than concentrating on removing the symptoms of illness, i.e. working against them, holistic healing considers symptoms to be the body's natural expressions and also as indicators of the right healing methods. In many cases when following a holistic healing treatment, symptoms get worse before they start to get better.

The Western understanding of illness

Today in the West we lack many of the foundations necessary for a full holistic understanding of illness and healing. This is partly because we have become accustomed to the workings of the human body being explained in purely biophysical terms, i.e. in terms of mechanical, physical and chemical facts which can be demonstrated scientifically. However, although scientific thought is superbly suited to explanations of technical processes, it fails to grasp the emotional and spiritual side of human existence.

Western emphasis on the physical

We should not make the mistake of applying purely scientific principles to essentially unscientific holistic healing methods. Rather we should seek to approach such forms of therapy with a new understanding. Just as the body-soul-spirit unit cannot be measured, or even proven to exist by scientific methods, a human being cannot be comprehended through scientific terms alone and a full understanding of human disorders requires more than an explanation of biophysical and chemical reactions.

Knowledge of people is important

Therapists rely as much on their understanding of people and human nature as on a knowledge of illnesses. However, as medical science delved deeper into the workings of the physical body, gaining understanding of its internal mechanisms right down to its smallest units, scientific explanations of medical problems came to the fore. This scientific approach led to the body being seen increasingly as an object, and if spiritual or emotional aspects were considered at all, it was often merely as functions of the physical body.

Criticism of this one-dimensional view, and doubts about its wisdom, are as old as medicine itself. Recently, however, such criticism has gone so far as to claim that traditional Western medicine, and the social development of which it is part, have both reached their natural limit. We are frequently made aware of Nature's destruction in the pursuit of human 'progress', and the danger to our surroundings is mirrored by a similar threat to the nature of human beings. The scientific method of dissecting in order to understand means that we no longer have a unified, holistic way of looking at people – of regarding a human being as a whole living unit.

The human being is a whole unit

To overcome the divisions and boundaries that face us today, many people feel we need to reassess where we are coming from, and what we are looking for. Most of the well-known, so-called "alternative" healing therapies, such as acupressure, have overcome these boundaries by looking back over thousands of years to ancient natural healing methods.

Basic principles of natural healing

Natural healing does not force something onto the body, because to do so could merely impose an additional burden. Instead, natural healing tries predominantly to make the body receptive to healing. This principle can be found in virtually all cultures. Every social community, every tribe, had rituals specifically for dealing with ill people which aimed to create a healing ambience. In practice, this principle largely translates into solidarity, trust, and a willingness to be open, to share, to help and not to judge.

Universal natural law

The holistic science of healing is an open system which builds from the assumption that we live in accord with Nature, which has made us as it has made all other forms of life. Therefore, in a normal situation, we can look after ourselves in a natural and effective way. Acupressure is a natural healing method using knowledge that has been defined by experience.

In accord with nature

In addition, there are four therapeutic principles which form the ground rules of every natural healing treatment:

Four basic principles

- the therapy must be natural;
- above all, the treatment must not be damaging;
- it must be holistic;
- it must stimulate and support the natural reactions of the body and the natural forces of healing.

Behind the first of these principles is the belief that only natural healing measures and substances can stimulate the natural reactions of the body, and so bring about lasting improvements in health without causing side-effects.

The second principle reflects a contrast with orthodox medicine which achieves a direct, measurable and quick effect, but often at the cost of unwanted side-effects. Natural medicine works on a more indirect level, achieving its healing effect through stimulating the body's own defence mechanisms and healing powers. Taken in the right dosages and following correct procedures, it is virtually unknown for a natural healing therapy to produce damaging side-effects.

Disorders affect the whole organism

The third principle means that no organ of the body can get sick in isolation. When a disorder occurs, it is always as part of a process affecting the whole organism and the healing process involves the whole organism in trying find its balance again. It follows from this that the cause and explanation for the disorder are not necessarily in the organ which displays the symptoms. In holistic practice and method, the therapist never excludes the view of the person as a whole human being and aims to help the patient to see the underlying reason behind the disorder.

The fourth principle emphasises that a natural therapy does not work *against* an illness, but rather it works *for* the patient using his or her own energies. In the first instance, the word "therapy" can be taken to refer not to a particular treatment, but to a certain attitude to, or way of thinking about, "health" and "illness".

Illness as a crisis of life

The holistic perspective views an individual's life as a process of continuing development, with illness representing an interruption of this development. In other words illness is always a crisis of life, a challenge, which looked at in this way makes sense.

This way of thinking has long been eclipsed in the West by the one-dimensional scientific, functional perception of the body. Modern natural healing methods are breaking through this scientific way of thinking to show how other ways of healing, inspired partly by ancient methods, can be understood in a modern context that is valid for us today.

The Chinese energy teachings

At the root of Chinese healing science is a special understanding of human beings and their relationship with their natural surroundings and with the universe. Although this may seem a very different foundation to that of our modern Western healing methods, if we look at early European medical history we find central themes that are very similar to the holistic Chinese viewpoint.

Also known in the West

The writings of Hippocrates, usually regarded as the father of Western medicine, clearly show that he placed great emphasis on observation of the whole person and on the effect of diet, occupation and climate. He favoured a natural approach to cures, with the use of few drugs, stating that "our natures are the physicians of our diseases".

Plato, the philosopher and contemporary of Hippocrates, expressed a similarly holistic attitude to medicine. The healing of much suffering, he believed, was beyond the knowledge of doctors because they did not regard the whole. His philosophy was that a part can only be healthy if the whole is healthy. He could have been writing today, rather than nearly 2,500 years ago, when he said that ignoring this was the biggest mistake made when treating the human body.

Such thoughts were gradually pushed aside by the development of theories which had both scientific and technical orientation. These in turn led to the human being becoming seen by many as a functional biological system, which could be repaired on a mechanical basis.

Different forms of energy The Chinese science of healing continues to follow a unified holistic concept in which natural healing comes from a system of energy and vitality. Chinese medical philosophy describes a dozen basic forms of energy, and roughly twice as many variants. The most important aspects of these within the human body are introduced below:

The Chinese energy teachings are statements of philosophy as well as medical theory. Chinese philosophy connects the outer world (the macrocosm) to the individual's life (the microcosm). The universe, the natural world and a person's surroundings all follow the same basic principles as the life of the individual himself. An important foundation of Chinese medical philosophy is harmony of the microcosm and the macrocosm.

All Chinese forms of treatment therapy are based on the theory that a person's life energy – the *Chi* – flows through a system of channels in the body. These channels are known as meridians (see page 28).

■ In a healthy body free from disorders, the *Chi* flows freely and regularly along the meridians and the two polar forces of Yin and Yang are in balance with one another (see page 16). If a "blockage" occurs in a meridian so that the *Chi* can no longer flow freely, the harmony between the Yin and Yang forces will be disturbed, with one or other of them getting the upper hand. This creates an imbalance in the person who, as a result, feels unwell and becomes ill. Only when the balance of the forces is re-established will the individual be healthy again.

Yin and Yang

Being healthy and being ill are not thought of as conditions, but as phases in an ongoing process known as the "balance of the flow". This process could be compared with riding a bicycle: while the bicycle is moving it is easy to maintain your balance, but when the bicycle slows down and stops it falls over.

In the *I–Ching*, a fundamental book of ancient Chinese thought sometimes called "The Book of Changes", it states:

Once Yin – Once Yang – That is the Tao.

The Tao is divinity, both the way to it and the goal itself; at the same time, it is the beginning and the end of everything, it is the infinite void and the source of all being. The Tao is symbolised by a full circle, while its Chinese character is made up from the symbols for head and foot. Together they symbolise the connection between heaven and earth, between thinking and doing, the unity of spirit and movement. The Tao cannot be described in words. In the *Tao-te-Ching*, perhaps the most famous work of ancient Chinese philosophy, Lao Tsu wrote:

The one who knows does not speak;
the one who speaks knows nothing.

Yin–Yang symbol

The complementary forces of Yin and Yang permeate every branch of Chinese thought. They make up all aspects of life and everything is considered to happen as a result of the balance between them. Yin is perceived as female, dark, passive and absorbing; it is Earth and is present in valleys and streams. Yang is

Yin–Yang: a balance of forces

perceived as masculine, light, active and penetrating; it is Heaven and is present in mountains. Neither can exist without the other and this is graphically represented in the Yin–Yang symbol. The black and white halves of the circle correspond to the poles, Yin and Yang, and stream from the Tao: there is no Yang without Yin and in every Yin there is Yang.

The unity of Yin and Yang can be seen all around us. Movement and stillness, day and night, are often thought of as contrasts or opposites, but in fact they belong together: there is no movement without stillness, and day is not feasible without night. This indivisible unity, this essential harmony, can be found everywhere – in food* and drink, in an individual's personality, or in the relationship of people living together as much as in thought.

■   A balanced proportion of Yin and Yang is the fundamental basis of a healthy body, soul and spirit – a healthy person. Imbalance of Yin and Yang is seen as the root of all disorders and illnesses.

The human condition depends on the maintenance of balance between Yin and Yang. Both poles naturally strive for unification and harmony. The general principle is that Yang (Heaven = energy) enlivens Yin, whereas Yin (Earth = material) preserves Yang. Neither is better or stronger than the other, just different, and both are essential to each other.

Constant balance of Yin and Yang

By recognizing these poles within us and the constant striving for harmony, we take an important step towards a better understanding of ourselves and the body-soul balance which is a prerequisite of well-being.

* Different foods are categorised as Yin or Yang. Yang nourishment contains more energy and can be stored longer; Yin nourishment spoils more easily. If exerting oneself physically, one generally needs more Yang food; for mental work Yin is more appropriate. The way in which foods are prepared is also important.

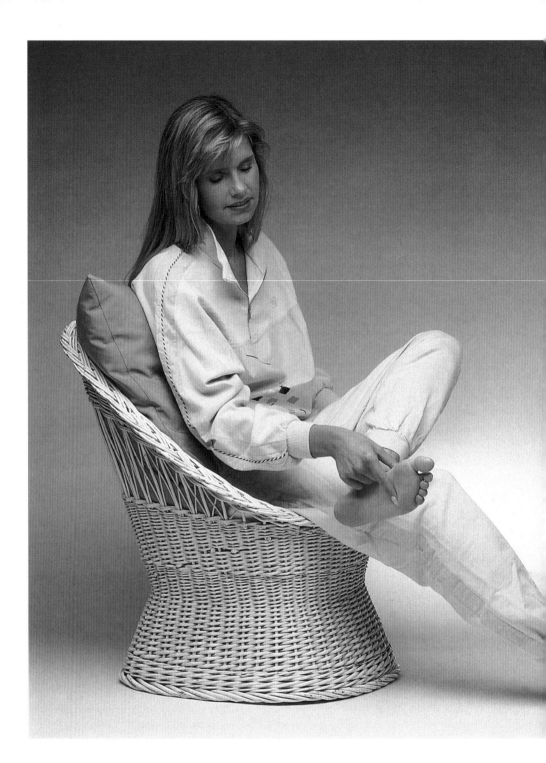

Natural healing with acupressure

Acupressure is a gentle Chinese
healing method which stimulates
the flow of energies in the body, thus
strengthening its self-healing powers.
The technique uses the application of
finger pressure at certain specific
points of the body to release built-up
energy and re-balance the body's
energy forces.

The effective use of acupressure
depends on applying the right amount
of pressure or grip and , most
importantly, on finding the right point
to press.

The essence and origins of acupressure

Acupressure = "point-pressure"

The word *acupressure* derives from the Latin words *acus*, meaning peak, needle or point, and *pressum*, meaning to press. The related technique of *acupuncture* derives its name from *pungere*, meaning to prick or sting. Acupressure and acupuncture share a common history: both healing methods developed out of ancient Chinese healing massage and the Chinese teachings on energy, and have a tradition stretching back thousands of years.

Ancient healing tradition

In acupressure, the body's energies are influenced and stimulated by finger – or in some cases thumb, or even foot – pressure at precise pressure points on the body. It is in essence a hand-treatment method, and as such has aspects in common with the Japanese form of massage called Shiatsu, which also stimulates vitality and whose name actually means "finger pressure".

In acupuncture the stimulation is created by the technique of inserting very fine gold, silver or stainless steel needles at one or more of over a thousand energy points on the body. As in acupressure, these points are situated along the body's energy channels (see pages 27–29), although acupuncture makes use of many more energy points than are used in acupressure.

To practise acupuncture requires specialist study and training in the precise locations, meanings and effects of each energy point. In contrast, acupressure is quite easy to learn: as a healing therapy it has been part of folk medicine in China for thousands of years.

Easy to learn

A short history of acupressure and acupuncture

Even though acupressure and acupuncture as they are practised today have descended from Chinese traditions, the use of similar techniques can be found in many cultures, indicating that their ultimate origins are probably much more widespread.

Original forms of acupressure

In China the techniques were synthesized into a system, but acupressure can be found in less rigid forms in all cultures, from so-called primitive tribes to modern technological societies. Some Bantu tribes have been reported to cure illnesses by scratching certain parts of the body, while a cannibal tribe of the Brazilian jungle was reputed to use blow-pipes to direct small arrows at precise parts of the body – a form of acupuncture. Investigations in various countries have found that children in pain will spontaneously press certain parts of the body which have nothing to do with – and are often distant from – the part that hurts.

We do not need scientific studies, however, to show us examples of instinctive acupressure. At some time, everyone will have found themselves fidgeting with their earlobe while deep in thought, or rubbing the bridge of their nose in tense or exhausting situations, or massaging their temples to soothe a headache. Drumming with the fingertips is as much an indication that one does not have energy as it is a sign of impatience.

Instinctive self-help

The principle of self-help through pressure can equally be observed in animals: if an animal has discomfort in an organ it may press itself against obstacles, or lie on top of branches or stones, to produce pressure on certain parts of its body and combat the pain.

Applies to humans and animals

■ All of this evidence leads to the conclusion that in its most basic form acupressure is a type of instinctive self-help used by both humans and animals.

The history of Chinese acupressure and acupuncture during the

Documented for thousands of years last 5,000 years has been documented from archaeological discoveries. Records preserved from the sixth century BC outline principles that are still largely valid today. Generally, the overriding system of energy points and methods of treatment have remained the same, while the underlying spiritual and philosophical foundation of the healing science have been moulded by ongoing cultural developments.

The development of acupressure and acupuncture

According to legend, the "Yellow Emperor" Huang Ti, who is reputed to have lived from 2698 to 2598 BC, first recognised and recorded the Chinese system of internal energies in the human body (although there is some evidence that the version in use today dates back only as far as the third century BC). This legendary ruler contributed a great deal to Chinese development as he is also said to have invented the wheel, systems of money, mathematics and astronomy, musical instruments and much more besides.

For a long time China was a complete mystery to Europeans. In the seventeen-hundreds missionaries returned to Europe bearing reports of Chinese culture and achievements, but attempts to introduce their methods of healing were not taken seriously. Even though Chinese techniques had a proven record of success stretching back thousands of years they were considered backward, and not all of China's acknowledged inventions – such as porcelain, paper, printing or gunpowder – could convince the Europeans that there might be something of substance in their medical knowledge.

Lack of understanding in West

Eventual introduction in Europe Although we know that acupuncture was used in England in the nineteenth century – it was reported as being of value in the treatment of pain in the first edition of the Lancet in 1823 – we know also that there was a cultural difficulty in getting across the validity of acupuncture and acupressure in Europe. The empirical

Europeans found it difficult to accept healing methods which, to them, were nothing short of mysticism. Language problems and translation errors further contributed to the generally sceptical reception given to both healing methods.

The interpretation of Chinese medicine in the West

The Chinese have developed a unique understanding of life – of nature, of people, of health and illness, and of the universe – that is difficult for those of us brought up in the West to comprehend. We have learned to believe only what can be proven scientifically, and in so doing have overlooked the fact that that laws of nature and the universe are valid, regardless of whether of not the human mind can comprehend them.

Science versus laws of nature

Using our scientific logic, it is impossible to grasp what a point on the big toe has to do with the pancreas – especially when we can find nothing to directly connect the point with the organ itself. We are used to regarding the human body first and foremost as physical material, whereas in Chinese healing science it is essentially an energy system made up of forces that work both for and against each other (see page 15). In such a system, the most important factor is to maintain balance between the forces, and once we comprehend this, acupressure becomes less of a mystery.

Acupressure seen the right way

With the recent rediscovery of the natural healing sciences and their potential for the treatment and prevention of illness, the healing methods of the Far East have gained new significance in the West.

Sensational successes in acupuncture were given much attention by the press. In 1971 an employee of the New York Times fell ill with appendicitis while in China. He was operated on in a Peking hospital under the influence of an acupuncture analgesic. Completely free from pain, he was fully conscious throughout and able to follow the progress of his own operation. Acupuncture

Indisputable eye-witness evidence

became instantly well-known in Austria in 1972 when a patient in Vienna was anaesthetized during a tonsil operation with only a few needles. These days, operations performed with acupuncture rather than general anaesthetic are no longer rare or even regarded with wonder.

Welcome collaboration

Medical practice in China today is a successful combination of modern medicine and traditional healing. There are some signs that in the West, too, collaboration is now growing between established traditional medicine and natural therapies. If such collaboration could be encouraged so that the two branches of medicine genuinely supplement each other, everyone concerned – doctors as well as patients – could only profit from this.

How does acupressure work?

For self-treatment with acupressure it is less important *how* the method works than the simple fact that it *does* work. However, the impressive successes of both acupuncture and acupressure have led many medical research institutes to investigate the reasons for their effectiveness. There has been much speculation and explanation, but as yet no theory has emerged that is entirely free of contradictions.

The first step: trusting the method

One argument often levelled at acupressure and acupuncture is that they only have a Placebo effect, i.e. that patients reporting improvement in their condition after treatment are in fact only reacting to the suggestion that treatment will bring improvement. This argument is easily contradicted, however, as both methods have been proven to work successfully in treating people who are unconscious and in treating animals. A patient cannot claim an improvement is due to treatment if they do not know they have had such treatment.

Carried out by an expert, acupuncture therapy can produce impressive results with many disorders, including: breathing and digestive organs; disorders of the nervous system and the bone and muscle structure. With the help of blood examinations, electrocardiograph methods (for measuring electrical activity in the heart) and spirometric methods (for measuring breathing), such successful treatments with acupuncture have been proven.

Successful treatments have been proven

It is recognised that the points on the body which are stimulated during acupressure and acupuncture do have a special energy or electrical capacity: at these points the conductive capabilities of the skin are greater than in the surrounding areas. Recently the opinion has also emerged that an "information system", running along the skin and in the body, forms itself at the embryonic stage of development, even before the central nervous system.

The nervous system is one of the most difficult areas of biology and medicine. Although much is still being discovered about it, the latest results of physiological research seem to be confirming the ancient teachings on the process and energy of life. The nerve fibres in the skin transfer many stimulants: electrical messages that travel down the nerves reacting to, for example, cold, heat or pressure. It is only in the brain that these will be identified as warmth, coolness or pain. Two types of nerve fibres are responsible for passing on stimulants to the brain: the first type pass all stimulants on slowly; the second pass on more powerful stimulants at top speed. If a very strong stimulant is passed on through a fast route, this will block the information from less pronounced stimulation. Thus the perception of pain can be prevented – which partially explains the success of acupuncture anaesthesia.

Passing on stimulants via nerve fibres

A Canadian scientist has proved that acupuncture and acupressure stimulate the production of the body's own natural painkiller, endorphins. These endorphins act just as intensively as the painkiller morphine. Further research projects concern themselves with electrical measurements of the skin's resistance, with the constitution of the tissue at the points of stimulation, and the influence of carrier substances in the brain.*

Production of the body's own pain- killers

* These carrier substances are neurotransmitters which pass on information from nerve cell to nerve cell. They influence everything which happens in an organism, both conscious and unconscious (instinctive) actions.

In Los Angeles the scientist H. Motoyama has been examining the routes of energy in the human body. His conclusion is that the life energies do not flow – as had been assumed – through the nervous system, but along their own physiologically provable channels. These channels are possibly synonymous with the previously mentioned information system which is now thought to form in the early embryo stage.

A project at the Herdecke Anatomical Institute in the University of Witten is researching into the morphology of acupuncture points, i.e. into the detail of their shape and form. The points are described as "specifically structured bundles" which penetrate the body's top layer of tendons, muscle and skin. As these represent particular anatomical structures and are located specifically in the area of acupuncture points, it is possible that they have a special function. Thus the most recent scientific medical research works towards confirming the validity of thousands of years of knowledge and practice.

Activating self-healing powers

■ The natural regeneration and healing capabilities of the body do not need scientific proof: everyone has observed these powers for themselves, from the healing of small cuts to large operation wounds and to recovery from broken bones and infectious disease. On the one hand we have forgotten how to deal with the self-healing powers of the body, and on the other we are not capable of supporting the self-healing energies because we no longer know the relevant procedures. But the self-healing powers are still there, and acupressure can help you to realise that again. It can activate the self-healing powers within us all – regardless of whether or not we can understand or approve the process.

About acupressure treatment

Before you begin there are some basic principles which you need to understand, as these will largely influence whether your self-help method is a success or failure.

In using acupressure as a natural healing method you are not treating the symptoms of a problem but the cause. According to Chinese belief, that cause is a disturbance in the balance of your vitality (see pages 16 and 30). Acupressure can help you re-establish the balance and restore harmony to the energy in your body.

Treating the cause of illness

■ Always keep in mind that you are not just using a technique: you are working with your body's own energies.

The energy channels in the body

The free flow of life's energy

The basis of Chinese healing science is the belief that it is not the trouble-free functioning of organs, bones, muscles and nerves that is most important for health, but the free, unhindered flow of life's energy, known as *Chi*.

This energy circulates in closed routes within the body and on the surface of the body. An illness occurs when the flow of energy along one or more of these routes is weakened or blocked – if an element gains the upper hand for any length of time over its neighbours, the harmonic balance of the body is broken. The reasons for such disturbances are diverse: they could be caused by the influence of the climate, by physical injuries, poor sustenance, or constant overwork.

It is the aim of acupressure to eliminate such disturbances in the flow of energy via certain points on the energy routes.

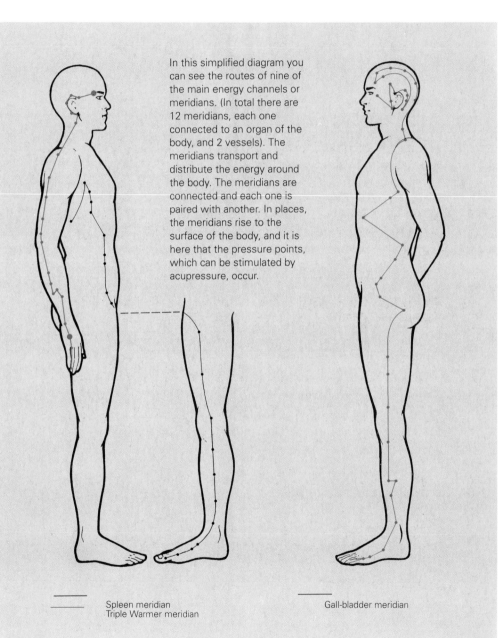

In this simplified diagram you can see the routes of nine of the main energy channels or meridians. (In total there are 12 meridians, each one connected to an organ of the body, and 2 vessels). The meridians transport and distribute the energy around the body. The meridians are connected and each one is paired with another. In places, the meridians rise to the surface of the body, and it is here that the pressure points, which can be stimulated by acupressure, occur.

Spleen meridian
Triple Warmer meridian

Gall-bladder meridian

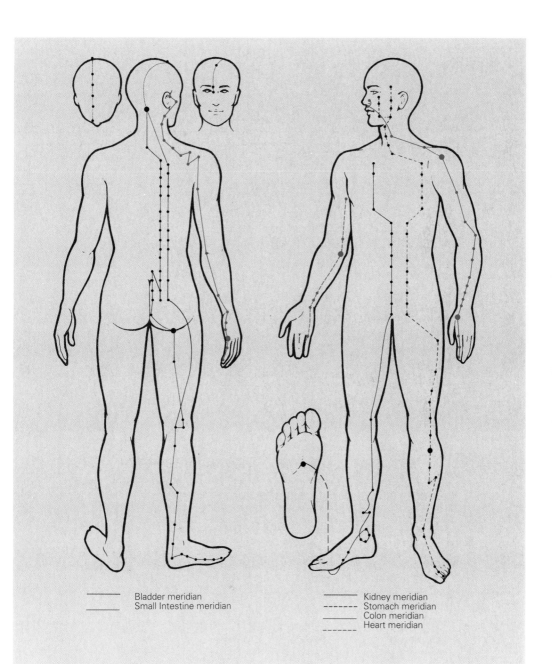

Bladder meridian
Small Intestine meridian

Kidney meridian
Stomach meridian
Colon meridian
Heart meridian

Balance of the energies Acupressure treatment essentially consists of restoring the energetic balance of the body. If a blockage has resulted in a build-up of energy, energy will be drawn off; if there is a lack of energy, energy will be supplied. The physical symptoms of the disorder are merely an indication to help identify which energy channels are unbalanced. Nearly all the points used in acupressure treatment are situated on the energy channels or meridians*. A few special points, which are to be found externally, are indicated on the diagrams on pages 28–29.

Variety of points and their effects

Compared to acupuncture, acupressure uses relatively few stimulation points. They are usually pressed with the tip of the index or middle finger or with the thumb (see page 32). The various points produce different reactions: stimulating certain points will produce a calming, sedative effect; stimulation of others **Calming or** will produce an activating, invigorating, tonic effect. The energy **invigorating** balance of your body, as reflected in its symptoms, dictates which **effect** type of point you should stimulate. The points of harmonisation are particularly suitable for preventative treatment. In Chinese medical theory, the following points are differentiated:

● **Points of harmonisation**
These are situated at the beginning and end of each energy channel. Their function is to harmonise the energies in all the related organs and groups of organs.

● **Points of stimulation (tonic points)**
On every energy channel there is only one point of stimulation which is able to mobilise energy and activity in the case of an energy deficiency. This particular treatment technique is called toning. Spare energy can also be released by stimulating these

* There are six Yin and six Yang meridians – located in pairs on the left and right sides of the body – and two vessels. Acupressure or acupuncture textbooks can provide more detail on the accurate routes of energy channels.

points. In Moxa Therapy (Moxibustion), the stimulation is brought about by burning little cones of medical herbs above the acupuncture point.

● **Calming points (sedative points)**
These points are treated whenever an excess or overflow of energy occurs, or if there is an imbalance in the relationship between tension and relaxation. Stimulation of the calming points has the effect of diverting energy.

● **Special points**
These are usually situated outside the meridians and have a strong effect on certain disorders.

● **Alarm points**
For those experienced in acupressure, these have a double function as both a diagnosis point and a first-aid point.

The treatment section of this book does not describe the individual points in detail. The points suggested for use are tried and tested, and an in-depth knowledge of energy science is not necessary for their successful application.

Finding the treatment points

For a successful treatment, it is important that you find the centre of each acupressure point you are using. The diagrams in the treatment section direct you to the general positions of the points relating to each symptom. From there, you must localise the actual point on your body using the sensitivity in your fingers.

Importance of sensitive fingers

"Feel" the difference Feel the pressure points with care and you will instinctively know when you hit the right spot. The tissue structure of the point often differs from the tissue surrounding it – you will feel a small inlet, or a slight change in the firmness of the tissue. Sometimes, under pressure, the right point will feel slightly more sensitive to pain than the surrounding area.

When treating a partner, please note:

All instructions for measurements using fingers, for example "finger width", always refer to the measurements of the person being treated, not the person doing the treatment.

Technical appliances There are some highly developed massage appliances on the market which can help in the location of acupressure points. They mainly function through recognising the electrical resistance of the skin in the point area. Usually they light up when they are above the point; in some a small massage device will automatically switch itself on. Although such appliances may be potentially attractive, they are expensive and are no replacement for the sensitive human hand.

The grip techniques

Next to every acupressure point in the treatment guide you will find instructions, in abbreviated form, on the appropriate grip technique to use in that particular treatment. The four main techniques used are described below.

Pressing

▶ **Pressing**

In the most common method of influencing the energy points you press the point with the tip of the index finger, middle finger or thumb. First press the fingertip to the centre of the point, then begin to massage in a clockwise, circling motion. Make two or three circling motions per second, moving around the point with firm skin contact. Points at the corners of a fingernail or toenail can be treated very effectively with the aid of an acupressure stick.   **The most common treatment technique**

● For acute pain or for a first treatment, press the points with gentle pressure, using circling massage.

● For chronic symptoms but otherwise good general condition, press with medium-strength pressure.

● Strong pressure with the thumb is only appropriate in certain cases, which are always indicated in the treatment instructions.

Tapping

▶ **Tapping**

Quick tapping of the treatment point with the tip of the index or middle finger.

Pushing

▶ **Pushing**

A pushing motion of the index or middle finger along one line of the meridian. The massaging finger should ideally be straight. Pushing can be done in two directions:

The direction determines the effect

● The proximal direction is towards the central part of a limb or the centre of the body. It has a strengthening, invigorating effect.

Parting

● The distal direction is away from the centre of the body to the outside or towards the extremities of fingers and toes. It has a softening and energy-diverting effect.

Merging

▶ **Parting and Merging**

This technique uses the thumbs in a pushing motion. In parting, the thumbs start together at the pressure point then push outwards. In merging, the thumbs come together directly over the point of treatment.

General rules for applying treatment

● You should not attempt acupressure when you are very tired, directly after meals, or after drinking alcohol.

Pay careful attention to the rules of treatment

● Treatment should be in a warm, well-aired room; warmth and fresh air have a relaxing effect.

● You need quiet: treatment should not be disturbed by television or radio, or by ringing telephones and door bells.

● Never attempt acupressure when you are feeling stressed.

About acupressure treatment

● Hands should be warm and clean and the fingernails should not be too long. Applying pressure with long fingernails could cause pain or even lead to injury.

● During treatment, focus on the thought that you are working with your life energies, rather than on the symptoms you are suffering from. The body's own regulatory powers should be at the centre of your attention.

● Do not press too many points too quickly – give your body time to process a given stimulation before moving on to another.

● Do not get impatient if there is no immediate success. With some points it can take up to 20 minutes after treatment before you will feel a reaction, such as an easing of pain or subsiding of symptoms.

Every person reacts differently

● Not all people react in the same way to acupressure on the individual points. Sometimes treatment of one point or combination of points may have the desired effect; at other times it may be a different combination which produces the best response. The sequences in which you treat the acupressure points come from experience and at first it will take time to discover the best combinations and orders. It is a good idea to record notes of the points which produced the desired reaction.

Duration of treatment

● The duration of the acupressure treatment varies from a few seconds up to 10 minutes, depending on the age and all-round energy situation of the individual being treated. In older people, energy blockages will have built up during the course of their lives, and these might take longer treatments to resolve. Small children, on the other hand, should be treated for only half a minute at the most. The duration given for treatments in this book should be regarded as guidance only.

● Whenever you feel that you want to stop the acupressure treatment of one particular pressure point, you should bring the entire treatment session to an end: this is the body's way of telling you that further stimulation cannot be absorbed and processed.

If you are not experienced with acupressure your energy system will be unfamiliar with this type of stimulation, and it may take a little while to notice the effect of the treatment.

Please note

Be aware of your reactions throughout the treatment. Stop the acupressure if you achieve a successful reaction, for example, if a pain eases off.

If a complaint in the treatment guide calls for the use of more than one acupressure point, the recommended duration of treatment represents the total acupressure time for the entire sequence. For example, if the recommended duration is two minutes for a sequence involving two pressure points, press each point for one minute.

If you experience unexpected physical disturbance – most likely a slight dizziness, because of too much pressure – simply stop the acupressure session. After a few moments you will feel better again.

● Usually, acupressure would be applied once or twice a day. Some points can be pressed more frequently according to the treatment needed, for example to ease a cold, cough or pains. Precise instructions accompany each complaint in the treatment guide.

● When treating another person the intensity of pressure is dictated by the person being treated. It is not important if the person giving the acupressure feels that he or she should apply a lot of pressure. Rather, the guide should be whether the receiving partner experiences the acupressure powerfully, and this does not necessarily depend on how powerful the pressure actually is.

Intensity of pressure

Treat both sides ● Nearly all acupressure points (apart from those on the "axis of symmetry") can be found as a mirror image on the left and right sides of the body: those on the right leg are mirrored on the left leg. Always press both points, and if possible press them at the same time, for example on both sides of the head or on both feet.

The potential and limitations of self-treatment

Acupressure does not produce miracles. When using acupressure as a self-treatment method you must always bear in mind its limitations as well as its potential for success.

• Acupressure does not cure every disorder, it does not work with every person, and it does not work at all times – even treatments you have successfully used before may not be so effective on another occasion.

Please note

When ill: see your doctor

Acupressure cannot replace orthodox medical treatment. If you are ill, you must consult a doctor. In certain cases, acupressure can provide useful support to conventional treatment: discuss any such treatment with your doctor.

• Acupressure is effective against disorders which have their origins in an imbalance of the body's energy. The techniques work towards a general harmonisation of the body's energy balance and the symptoms – the body's signals – become superfluous when balance is achieved.

• Acupressure is particularly effective: in the treatment of pain; for general relaxation; in treating emergencies (until medical help is available); as a preventative health measure; for harmonising and balancing tension; for the promotion of well-being.

Good for treating pain

• Acupressure has a strong balancing effect on the nervous system. Many complaints have their origins in various malfunctions of the nervous system: one estimate by orthodox medical practitioners put the figure as high as two-thirds of total health problems.

■ The treatment section of this book (see pages 44–92) concentrates on disorders which respond well to self-treatment.

**Important:
the
confident
diagnosis**

Treating yourself demands a responsible approach and requires a confident diagnosis. The true role of acupressure is in the preservation and maintenance of health. Before the detailed treatments for disorders, there are instructions for simple preventative acupressure treatments which can be included in your daily routine to help keep your health trouble-free (see page 42).

■ If you ever begin to feel unwell during acupressure treatment, simply stop the treatment. The treatment should also be stopped if the symptoms become worse. These are both exceptional circumstances which are very unlikely to occur if you follow the treatment rules carefully. Used properly, acupressure can bring about a noticeable improvement in symptoms fairly quickly; with patience, disorders will often clear up completely.

**Stop any
treatment if
it produces
discomfort**

Please note

Important

You must not use acupressure treatment in the following circumstances:

● If you have an acute organic heart complaint or circulation disorder.

● If there is skin or tissue damage around the treatment points, such as an open or festering wound, a cut or bruise, a fungal infection, or inflammation.

● During pregnancy certain pressure points should not be used. If you are pregnant, before commencing any treatment discuss it with a doctor who has experience of natural remedies and acupressure.

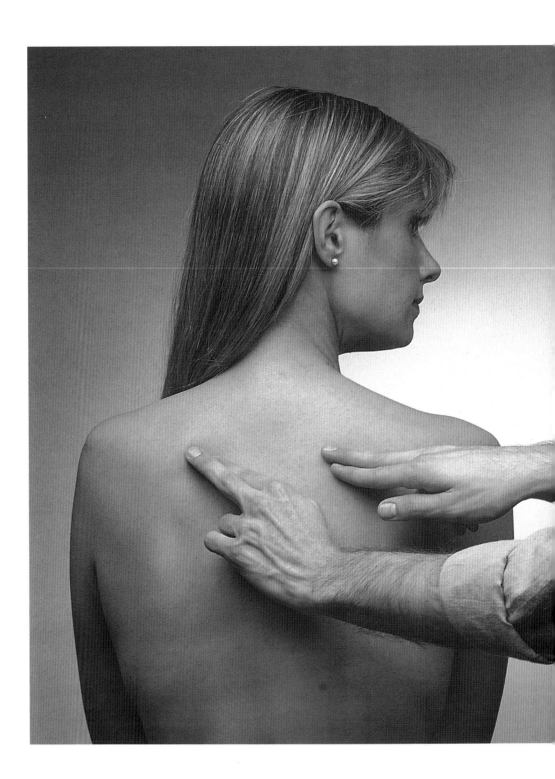

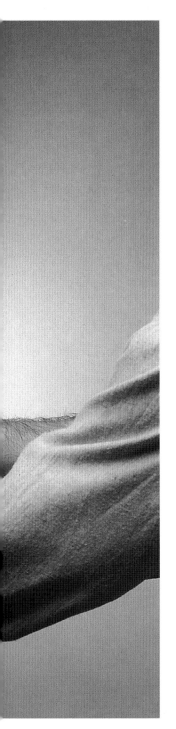

Acupressure made easy

All kinds of everyday complaints, as well as the symptoms of many chronic conditions, can be effectively treated through acupressure. Treatment needs patience, however, and you should not expect immediate results. It is also important to realise that acupressure cannot cure everything.

To achieve the best results with acupressure, you should relax and be honest with yourself about your symptoms and what your body is feeling. The techniques outlined in this guide will help you to harmonise the energies in your body. The methods are gentle and very safe: the only "damage" that can happen to you during treatment is that you do not feel anything.

Preparation before practice

This section describes how to put selected acupressure techniques into practice to alleviate common complaints. Many uncomfortable and painful disorders respond well to self-treatment with acupressure. The guidelines and instructions which are given take into account the proven capabilities of acupressure as well as its limitations as a self-treatment therapy.

The complaint descriptions

Complaint descriptions and treatments

The complaints are listed alphabetically under their familiar names. There is a detailed description of the symptoms, followed by precise instructions for the recommended acupressure treatment.

● The location of the pressure points used in each treatment are clearly indicated in the diagrams. Instructions on the particular technique to be applied in each case, the intensity of pressure and the duration of treatment are given below each diagram. See pages 32-33 for further details of treatment techniques.

> *Please note*
> The time given for each treatment is indicated below each pressure point diagram. This only apply when it is the only point used in the treatment. If the treatment involves acupressure on a sequence of points, the total combined treatment time should not exceed the time recommended.

● The descriptions may indicate that other, similar health disorders should also be treated – either with acupressure or with other natural healing methods. If you follow all the recommendations, you could speed up the healing process.

● In some cases treatment recommendations are given for complaints that do not require a detailed description. These disorders can be found in the index on pages 93-94, which lists all of the complaints dealt with in the book.

● The selected self-treatment points are easily accessible and have proved successful in practice. The Chinese have given all the acupressure points figurative and, in some cases, poetic names. Here, the names are represented by English translations of the Chinese terms.

Before starting any treatment, go through the rules for treatment listed below and on page 33 to make sure that everything possible is done to facilitate the success of the treatment.

Treatment rules

● Make sure you are not tired and have not just eaten, or drunk alcohol.
● The treatment room should be warm and well ventilated.
● You should have peace, quiet and plenty of time.
● Your hands should be clean and warm and your fingernails short.
● The part of the body to be treated should be supported on a strong and stable base.
● Focus all your attention on what you are doing: harness your life energies to promote the healing.
● Press one point on the right side of the body, then the equivalent point on the left side, then wait calmly for the body's reaction.
● Observe your body's reactions closely: this will tell you the order in which you should treat the points.

● The intensity of pressure depends on what you feel. If a partner is doing the treatment, the person receiving treatment must determine the intensity of pressure.
● The treatment duration indicated is the maximum treatment time for anyone new to acupressure.
● If you use a particular acupressure massage regularly over a period of time you may find that you become more receptive towards that particular stimulation. If you feel this happening, you can cut the duration of treatment at the affected acupressure points by anything from 15 to 30 seconds.
● End the treatment as soon as you feel that you should stop, or when the person you are treating wants you to stop. Learn to trust the signals of the body.

Preventative care

The main concern of Chinese health care is to maintain a person in good health, i.e. the practice of preventative medicine. Even if you do not have a specific complaint that you want to treat, acupressure can still be of great benefit to you as a means of maintaining your well-being. These two pages describe some techniques which can help keep your body's energies in balance, thus ensuring that major energy disturbances do not occur and cause illness.

Stimulating the circulation of energy

One preventative technique is acupressure at the "points of harmonisation". These are located at the beginning and end of each energy channel or meridian. By pressing these points you encourage the constant circulation of

energy, and enable your system to compensate for any minor irregularities in the overall energy balance.

Treatment

▶ The harmonisation points are at the corners of the fingernails and toenails.

● With the tip of a finger, press each of these points on your hands and feet for about one minute.

● Make time for this treatment two or three times a week.

Strengthening the Yin and Yang energies

Another simple preventative method involves stimulating the Yin and Yang energy potential. Yin energy controls matter, which includes your body, while Yang energy controls the flow of energy through the body. The relationship could be compared to that of a horse and its rider, with Yin being the horse and Yang the rider. Only when Yin and Yang are in balance will you feel healthy.

Yang energy regulates both activity and stillness. If the

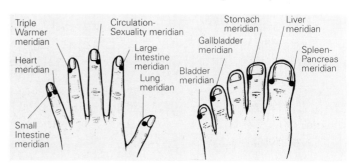

Triple Warmer meridian
Circulation-Sexuality meridian
Heart meridian
Large Intestine meridian
Lung meridian
Small Intestine meridian
Stomach meridian
Gallbladder meridian
Bladder meridian
Liver meridian
Spleen-Pancreas meridian

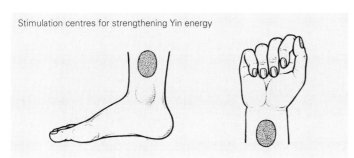
Stimulation centres for strengthening Yin energy

body's Yang energy controls the Yin energy correctly, the body's energy will be balanced and available where it is needed. In phases of relaxation, you will feel calm and restful.

Acupressure applied to Yin energy centres produces "matter-enhancing" effects which support the build up of physical strength. To improve control of your body's energies and optimise the Yang principle in your make-up, press those parts of the body which access your Yang energies. This will also strengthen your mental capacity.

Treatment

▶ Yin energy
On the underside of your forearms just above the wrists, and on the inside of your legs just above the ankles, are the stimulation centres which influence the Yin energies of the body.

● With gentle pressure, rub these centres, one after the other, until they are warm. On the forearms, use the finger surface or knuckles of a lightly closed fist. Do this every morning just after waking up.

▶ Yang energy
There are three stimulation centres for Yang energy and our mental and spiritual powers. Try them all out and see for yourself which one is most effective for you. The stimulation centres are located: (1) at the lower end of the breastbone; (2) on the side of your forearm just above the wrist; and (3) behind the ear lobe. By stimulating these centres, you can promote the development of your mental capacity.

● Rub your chosen Yang area, or areas, both in the morning and evening. You can try using a few drops of Hypericum oil (also knows as St John's wort oil) for your morning massage and a few drops of Sylmarin or milk thistle oil in the evening. St John's wort oil helps in the regulation of activity and is particularly suitable for daytime use, while milk thistle oil promotes calmness and is suited to night use.

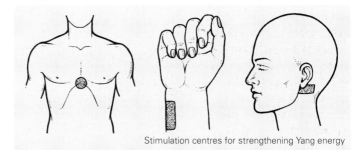
Stimulation centres for strengthening Yang energy

An A to Z of complaints and their treatments

Anxiety attacks

Anxiety attacks often occur without any obvious reason. Physical symptoms include perspiration, spasmodic chest pains, difficulty breathing, restlessness, impairment of motor skills, dizziness, and insomnia.

■ If you suffer regularly from anxiety, consult your doctor.

Anxiety attacks can be linked to many symptoms which occur without the existence of an organic, physical disorder. However, many of the "emotional" symptoms linked with anxiety attacks, such as despondency, melancholy and lack of motivation, which are commonly thought of as signs of depression, can be caused by a number of physical disorders. It is important that these symptoms are also treated.

■ It is advisable to support the recommended acupressure treatment with additional natural preventative measures, including a high-quality diet, herbal teas, relaxation, and breathing exercises. Together, these measures can harmonise your psychological balance, thus removing the cause of the anxiety attacks.

Treatment

▶ Do not expect this acupressure treatment to work overnight. Work through the points calmly and regularly and observe your reactions over a period of 2 to 3 weeks.

Please note

In cases of depression, never press points which have a calming effect.

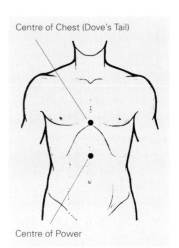

Centre of Chest (Dove's Tail)

Centre of Power

● Centre of Chest (= balancing energy point). Press up to 4 times daily with the middle finger, with changing pressure, in the direction of the neck – medium to strong pressure, 5–7 minutes.

● Centre of Power (halfway between the navel and the end of the breastbone) in combination with Divine Gate zone (see page 45) and Centre of Chest. Press – medium pressure, 3 minutes.

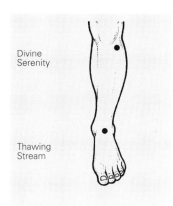

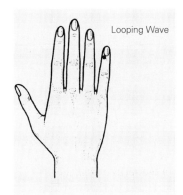

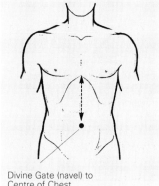

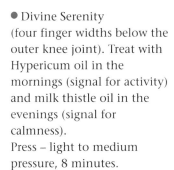

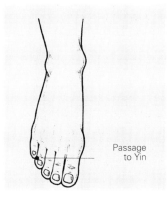

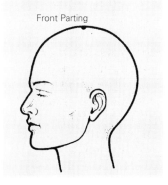

● Divine Serenity
(four finger widths below the outer knee joint). Treat with Hypericum oil in the mornings (signal for activity) and milk thistle oil in the evenings (signal for calmness).
Press – light to medium pressure, 8 minutes.

Acupressure of the Divine Serenity point balances the energies in the autonomic nervous system to make us more relaxed and able to cope with the strains of daily life. The name indicates how strong the effect of this point can be.

● Thawing Stream
(= invigorating point).
Press – medium pressure, 5 minutes.

● Looping Wave
(= invigorating point).
Press – strong pressure, 3 minutes.

● Passage to Yin
(= invigorating point).
Press – strong pressure, 5 minutes.

● Divine Gate (navel)
to Centre of Chest.
Push – gentle pressure, 5 minutes.

● Front Parting
(three finger widths in front of the crossing point of a line running over the centre of the head and a line between the top of the ears).
Press – gentle pressure, 3–5 minutes.

Appetite loss

Loss of appetite is usually a temporary disturbance. If it persists, however, it might be a sign of a more serious problem, for example, the start of an infectious disease.

■ If loss of appetite persists, consult your doctor.

Children often experience a change in their appetite pattern as part of their natural growth and development. Short periods of appetite loss can be a natural reaction, for example, to an upset in the digestive system. Other problems, such as difficulties at school, could also lead to a lack of appetite in children. However, if the child's body weight drops dramatically (to 20 per cent under average) he or she must be examined by a doctor. When the body is underweight its immune system is weakened, making the individual far more prone to physical disorders, such as colds and flu. Anorexia in adolescence is caused by emotional problems, which may require psychotherapy.

Treatment

▶ Acupressure is especially effective in cases where the cause of the appetite loss is psychological. It can reactivate the natural controlling mechanisms of the appetite. The best time for treatment is about 20 minutes before meals.

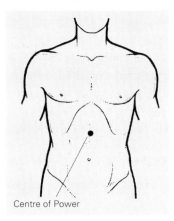
Centre of Power

● Centre of Power
(on the midline of the body, halfway between the navel and the end of the breastbone). This point is particularly suitable if the cause of appetite loss is psychological.
Press (from below upwards) – gentle pressure,
3 minutes.

● Looping Wave

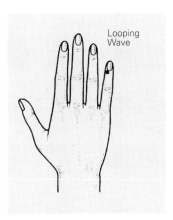
Looping Wave

(on the nail bed of the little finger). Press – strong pressure, 5 minutes.
● Inner Gate
(below the wrist).
Press – gentle pressure,
5–7 minutes.

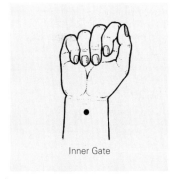
Inner Gate

Breathing

Backache

Tension in the muscles in the back and spine, damage caused by wear and tear of the vertebrae, often caused by sitting in the same position for hours on end at work, can lead to chronic backache in many cases.

■ It is important to see your doctor if you have chronic backache so that irreparable spine damage can be prevented.

The Treatment

▶ Acupressure has a harmonising effect on the toxicity of the muscular system. A general relaxation of the back muscles can be achieved via the special point KA-TE. This further relieves the nerve ends at the vertebrae.

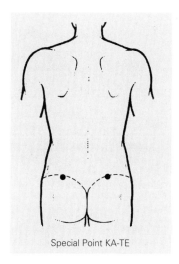

Special Point KA-TE

● Special Point KA-TE (left and right, directly above the pelvis bone). Use the help of a partner. Press/part – gentle to medium pressure, 10 minutes.

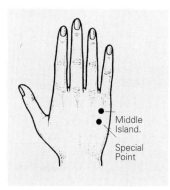

Middle Island.

Special Point

● Middle Island. Press – strong pressure, 5 minutes.

● Special Point (directly behind the ankles, one finger width behind the point, Middle Island). Especially effective for backache caused by bending. Press – strong pressure, 5 minutes.

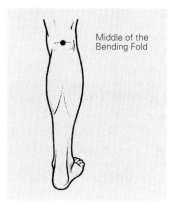

Middle of the Bending Fold

● Middle of the Bending Fold. Press – gentle pressure, 3 minutes.

Bedwetting

The cause of this weakness of the bladder is as likely to be psychological as physical.

When children wet the bed: If there is no physical problem causing the child to wet the bed, then the syndrome usually signals a means of releasing psychological pressure. Punishments, threats and accusations will only make the problem worse, but a simple acupressure technique can help to stop the bedwetting. Children who are old enough to understand can be taught the technique as a self-treatment.

Possible reasons for the child's stress – for example, a difficult situation within the family or at school – should be looked into and dealt with.

If the child also wets himself or herself during the day, this often points to a physical cause, such as an infection of the kidneys or urinary tract. In this case, consult your doctor.

When adults wet the bed: A prolonged bladder disorder may herald the beginning of a nervous condition. Consult your doctor.

Please note
In regular treatment, after a period of time it is best to press all three points daily for 3 minutes before going to bed.

Treatment

▶ Treatment of the following acupressure points can balance the psychological energies and normalise the tension of the bladder muscles.

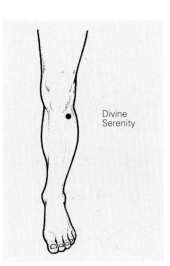

Divine Serenity

● Divine Serenity.
Press – medium pressure, 5-10 minutes.

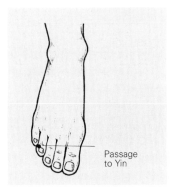

Passage to Yin

● Passage to Yin.
Press, with sideways pressure towards the big toe – light building to strong pressure, 5 minutes.

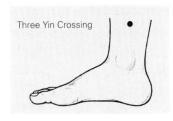

Three Yin Crossing

● Three Yin Crossing (four finger widths above the highest point of the inner ankle).
Press towards the knee – press/part, light building to medium pressure, up to 10 minutes.

Bladder problems

The ability to retain urine is controlled by tension of the muscular system. Lack of bladder control resulting in urinary dribbling can be due to weak muscle tone in the bladder muscle. However, bladder function is also closely related to a person's psychological state of health: most people have experienced extreme moments of tension or fear which has resulted in difficulty controlling the bladder. If there is a problem with bladder function, therefore, it is important that it is looked at in close connection with the person's psychological condition.

Treatment

▶ Depending on the nature of the problem, the bladder muscles could need to be strengthened in order to increase control, or relaxed in order to ease off muscle tension. Acupressure can be used in either case, and can also be used to help prevent a chill on the bladder turning into cystitis.

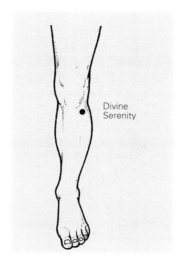

● Divine Serenity – for general harmonisation. Press – medium pressure, 5-8 minutes.

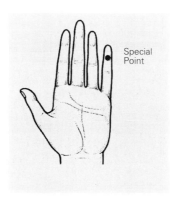

● Special Point (on the little finger, in the first crease). Press – strong pressure, 30 seconds.

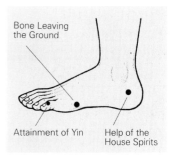

To aid retention of urine:
● Bone Leaving the Ground (in the hollow of the middle foot bone before the joint of the small toe). Press – strong pressure, 3-5 minutes.
● Attainment of Yin. Press – medium pressure, 5 minutes.

For urinary dribbling :
● Help of the House Spirits (on the outside of the foot directly on the heel bone) with Attainment of Yin Press – medium pressure, 5-10 minutes.

■ A fairly common cause of bladder problems is the presence of bladder stones. If the treatment does not improve the condition, consult your doctor about possible physical causes.

High blood pressure

About ten per cent of people suffer from high blood pressure. The condition rarely produces symptoms: it is usually only diagnosed if you visit the doctor for a check-up for other reasons.

In high blood pressure the systolic pressure, i.e. the higher of the two blood pressure measurements, is always over 140 mm Hg. It is the result of a contraction of the vascular system which demands a higher performance of the heart-rate.

Causes of high blood pressure include natural predisposition, infections, hormonal disorders, allergies and poor or inappropriate diet. Side-effects include headaches, dizziness, buzzing in the ears, frequent irritability, a feeling of "being under pressure" and insomnia. People who are overweight are particularly at risk. If you have high blood pressure, you have an increased risk of suffering a heart attack.

Treatment

▶ Acupressure can provide effective support to the medical treatment of high blood pressure.

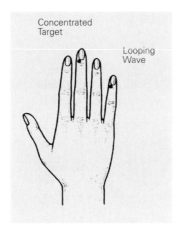

● Concentrated Target with Looping Wave (= harmonisation points on the nail beds of the middle and little fingers). These points can be repeatedly acupressed daily.
Press – medium pressure, 5 minutes.

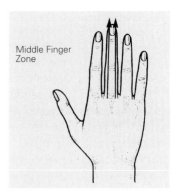

● Middle Finger Zone Achieves an energy-building effect through pulling the finger "longer" with the thumb and index finger of the other hand.
Push towards the fingertip, 5 times each per hand, several times a day.

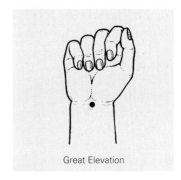

● Great Elevation (= calming point; in the middle of the wrists, directly behind the carpal bone).
Press – medium pressure, 5 minutes.

Low blood pressure

Low blood pressure is not considered a health problem in this country. Many people live with it without suffering any complaints or symptoms, and because the condition reduces pressure on the vascular system, the life expectancy of people with low blood pressure is, on average, higher than that of people with normal blood pressure results.

However, in some cases low blood pressure causes headaches and dizziness, a lack of energy, severe tiredness and a greater need for sleep. One of the best things for the condition is movement to stimulate the circulation. Alternating hot and cold showers is also advisable. In low blood pressure the systolic measurement is under 100 mm Hg.

Treatment

▶ Acupressure can help to stimulate the circulation and relieve the effects of low blood pressure.

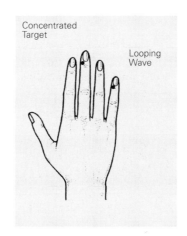

● Concentrated Target with Looping Wave.
These points can be pressed repeatedly during the day, if required.
Press – medium to strong pressure, 5 minutes.

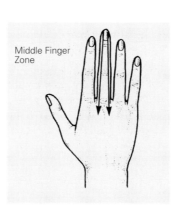

● Middle Finger Zone. Push towards the wrist, 5 times each hand, several times a day.

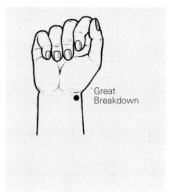

● Great Breakdown (on the wrist line, under the ball of the thumb, on the extension of the index finger). Press – medium pressure, 5 minutes.

problems

In holistic teachings breath is synonymous with life itself and it is of great importance in natural health care. There are many causes of breathing problems and they can be as much psychological as physical. If under normal conditions – i.e. not straight after physical exertion – you are short of breath, breathe unnaturally fast, or wheeze a lot, acupressure may help.

The onset of a spasm of breathing trouble can be anything from a feeling of apprehension to a complete tensing up of the bronchial muscles. If you suffer from breathing problems, get to know your stress level, and do not be afraid to ask others to modify their behaviour if it provokes a problem. If, for example, cigarette smoke affects you, then say so.

■ To check if your breathing is healthy, try this simple test: you should be able to fill a plastic bag measuring 15 x 25 cm with just one out-breath.

Treatment

▶ The following acupressure techniques can reduce the frequency of asthma attacks.

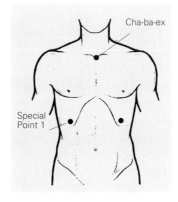

● Cha-ba-ex
(a special point at the top of the breastbone in the hollow of the collarbone joint). Press in an upwards direction (can also be tapped) – gentle pressure increasing to medium, 5–10 minutes.
● Special Point 1
(midway vertically between the chest and navel, in a line directly below the nipples). Press with the middle finger in a strong circular motion, 5–10 minutes.

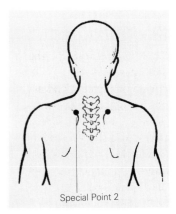

Special Point 2

● Special Point 2
(two finger widths to the left and right of the spine, level with the third vertebra). With the help of a partner: press/part – starting gently, 5–10 minutes.

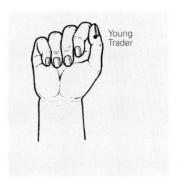

Young Trader

● Young Trader
(= masterpoint of the lung). Press – strong pressure, 5 minutes.

Circulation problems

Cold hands and feet signal a disturbance of the circulatory system and are often a sign of the onset of illness. A well-functioning circulation supplies the whole body with vitamins and nutrients. Eating a good diet and taking regular exercise to stimulate the circulation are vitally important if you want to keep your circulatory system healthy. A regular exercise programme can also balance any pressures of your work. Try to keep your weight within the average for your height and build, and avoid excessive consumption of alcohol. Statistically, more than half of peripheral circulatory disturbances are linked to smoking, so if you do smoke, try to give up.

■ There are many causes of circulatory problems. If you have a circulation disorder, consult your doctor to determine exactly what is causing the problem.

Treatment

▶ Acupressure helps to normalise any over-tense condition affecting the vascular system.

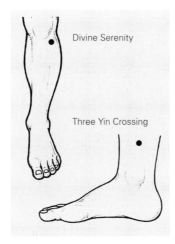

Divine Serenity

Three Yin Crossing

● Divine Serenity with Three Yin Crossing. Ideally, press on the left and right sides at the same time. Press – strong pressure, 10-15 minutes.
● Three Yin Crossing (four finger widths above the highest point of the inner ankle). Press/merge – start gently and build to medium pressure, up to 10 minutes.

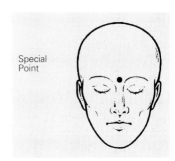

Special Point

● Special Point (between the eyebrows). Particularly for dizziness. Press – strong pressure, 5 minutes.

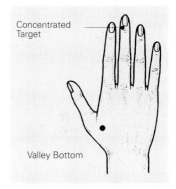

Concentrated Target

Valley Bottom

● Concentrated Target (= invigorating point). Especially for heart rhythms, press the points of both hands one after the other. Press – strong pressure, in a pulse-like rhythm, 1 minute per hand.
● Valley Bottom. Press, in direction of elbow – strong pressure, up to 10 minutes.

Colds

Colds are generally infections due to mild hypothermia of the body. Symptoms include light fever, headache, inflammation of the upper breathing passages, sore throat, and possibly also a stomach or intestinal disorder.

Treatment

▶ Acupressure treatment is directed towards building up the body's resistance and mobilising its defences against the cold infection. It cannot cure the infection, but it can help to relieve the symptoms and side-effects such as tiredness, pressure in the head and a blocked nose, thus easing the discomfort of the illness.

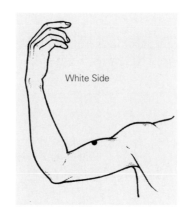

● White Side (in the middle of the upper arm, at the level of the biceps). Press – gentle pressure, 2-3 minutes.

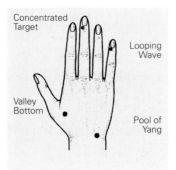

● Concentrated Target and Looping Wave. Press – mainly in times of high risk of infection – strong pressure, 3-5 minutes.
● Valley Bottom. Press – strong pressure, 5 minutes.
● Pool of Yang. Press – medium pressure, up to 10 minutes.

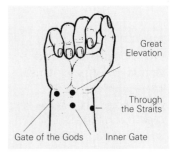

● Gate of the Gods. Press – medium pressure, 3-5 minutes.
● Great Elevation. Press – medium pressure, 3-5 minutes.
● Through the Straits. Grip round the wrist and press with the thumb and index finger. Press – strong pressure, up to 10 minutes.
● Inner Gate (three finger widths below the wrist). Press – medium pressure, 5 minutes.

Cold/hay fever

A cold is a symptom of many, often unspecified, viral infections. But it also has to do with the psychological condition – weakened resistance.

Hay fever is an allergic illness. It usually begins to develop during childhood and can lead to disorders of the bronchial tubes or even asthma. When the pollen count is high, three series of treatment methods per day can be used for prevention.

A cold can affect the sinuses. The mucus, which has been produced by the inflamed mucous membrane, can also create inflammation in the throat and can lead to coughing (see page 57 and page 74).

Treatment

▶ Acupressure can soothe a cold and ease the symptoms.

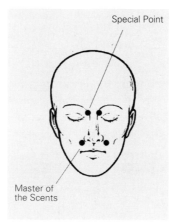

Special Point

Master of the Scents

● Special Point.
Treats infections in the nose and throat area. Press – gentle pressure, 5 minutes.
● Master of the Scents.
Has a harmonising effect, stimulates the circulation and makes the swelling of the mucous membrane fade. Press – gentle pressure, 5 minutes.

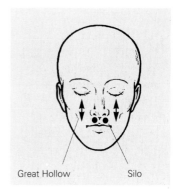

Great Hollow   Silo

● Great Hollow.
Push – 3 minutes.
● Silo.
Press – medium pressure, 5 minutes.

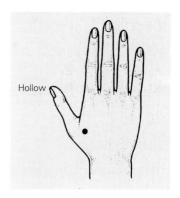

Hollow

● Hollow.
Has the same effect as Master of the Scents. Press/push – medium pressure, if necessary several times a day, 2 minutes.

Constipation

Apart from infections of the intestines, function disorders of the adjoining thyroid glands, wrong nutrition or potassium deficiency, constipation may be caused by psychological problems. According to the wholesome science of healing, people who suffer from constipation are extremely tidy, they are withdrawn and they are very much governed by performance. Constipation can also be due to laziness of the intestines. A person with a well-functioning digestive system should normally have one bowel movement a day.

■ Take regular exercise and adjust your diet so that it includes plenty of roughage. Laxatives should only be taken in consultation with your doctor, because your bowels could get accustomed to them (see also stomach and intestine disorders, pages 85-86).

Treatment

▶ Acupressure helps bowel movements become regular.

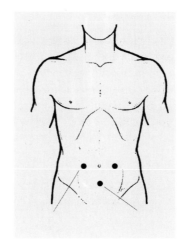

● Heaven's Axis.
Press – gentle pressure, 2-4 minutes.
● Sea of Energy.
Press – medium pressure, 5 minutes.

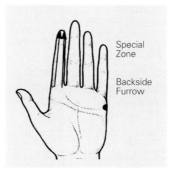

● Special Zone
(on the index finger).
Acupress both the left and right hand. Push towards fingertips – 10 times each.

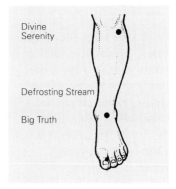

● Backside Furrow.
Press – strong pressure, 5 minutes.
● Divine Serenity.
Loosens cramp in the intestine muscles (also 3 miles, page 79). Press – strong pressure, 10 minutes.
● Defrosting Stream.
Press – medium to strong pressure, 5 minutes.
● Big Truth.
Press – medium pressure, 5 minutes.
● In addition acupress the Great Hollow point (page 55).

Coughs

Coughing is a natural reflex of the body to free itself of harmful substances in the breathing area. Anything that disturbs the breathing passages – foreign bodies, dust, phlegm, infection, smoking – creates an urge to cough. Severe fits of coughing are separated by cramp-like gasps for air. Coughing is a natural self-help mechanism of the body. Medications that stifle coughing should therefore be taken with care.

■ A cough can be a sign of more serious illness. If you feel stabbing pains in the chest when you cough, you should seek advice from a doctor. Likewise, if you see traces of blood in any phlegm you cough up, or if your cough persists longer than two to three weeks, see your doctor.

Treatment

▶ Acupressure can soothe the irritated mucous membrane of the throat. When using the treatment during a coughing fit, try to breathe deeply and slowly.

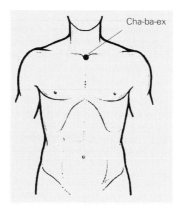

● Cha-ba-ex
(at the top of the breastbone in the hollow of the collar-bone joint). For a severe coughing fit press this point with the thumb or index finger, using strong constant pressure and a rotating motion. Press – strong pressure, 5 minutes.

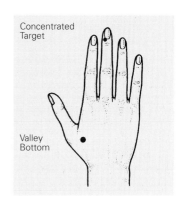

● Concentrated Target. Press – medium pressure, 5 to 10 minutes.
● Valley Bottom. Press – strong pressure, 5 minutes.

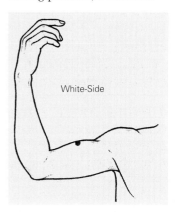

● White-Side
(in the middle of the upper arm, at the level of the biceps). Treat only for 30 seconds to soothe the urge to cough. Press/distribute – gentle pressure, 1-2 minutes.

Diarrhoea

There are many causes of diarrhoea: poor diet, infection, inflammation, metabolic disorder, the intake of certain medicines, tension or psychological stress. Severe diarrhoea results in loss of body fluids and minerals. These losses need to be made up, either by drinking unsweetened herbal tea with salt, or a special rehydration solution which can be obtained from the chemist.

■ Diarrhoea can be acute (short-lived), chronic (lasting a few days or longer), or can occur intermittently with breaks in between bouts. Mild bacterial diarrhoea will disappear on its own after a short time, but in cases of chronic diarrhoea the cause should be investigated and diagnosed by a doctor.

Treatment

▶ Diarrhoea caused by psychological stress (for example nervousness before an exam, or a frightening situation), responds well to acupressure. Treatment can also help with intestinal cramps and irritation of the intestinal membrane

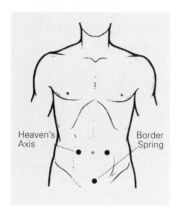

● Heaven's Axis
(3 finger widths to the right and left of the navel).
Press/merge – medium pressure, 3 minutes.
● Border Spring
(one hand's width above the pubic bone).
Press/merge – medium pressure, 5 minutes.

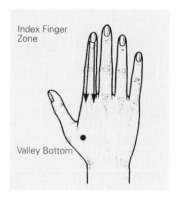

● Index Finger Zone.
Push sideways, towards the base joint, several times daily, up to 2 minutes.
● Valley Bottom.
Press – strong pressure, up to 10 minutes.

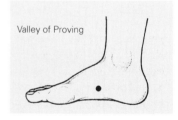

● Valley of Proving
(above the centre of the foot instep).
Press – medium pressure, 5 minutes.

Elbow pains

The immediate cause of elbow pain is usually strain or overexertion through awkward or repetitive movement. Certain types of sport or work can cause irritation or infection in the area of the joint connected to the sinews and muscles of the forearm. The resulting painful condition is commonly known as tennis elbow. Problems with the cervical vertebrae are also often connected to elbow pains (see spinal cord problems, page 83).

Acute tennis elbow can lead to calcium deposits on the bone, painful changes in the joint ligaments and nervous pains. Thorough examination and treatment should be sought from a doctor. Acupressure can effectively assist prescribed treatment to deal with any infection and to help dampen the pain.

■ If you suffer from elbow pains, a doctor or orthopaedic practitioner should diagnose the cause.

Treatment

▶ The acupressure treatment focuses on a point within the painful area.

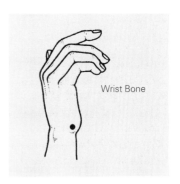

● Wrist Bone.
Press towards elbow – strong pressure, 5-10 minutes.

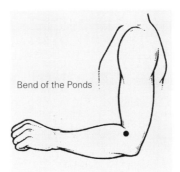

Bend of the Ponds

● Bend of the Ponds (at the crease above the joint when the arm is bent).
Press – medium pressure, 10 minutes.
The best method is to rest the painful elbow in the open hand of the other arm and press with the middle finger. At the same time make gentle turning movements with the hand of the painful arm, as if it were a key.

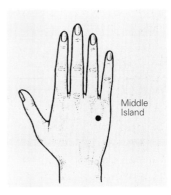

Middle Island

● Middle Island (between the outer two bones on the back of the hand).
Press – strong pressure, 5-10 minutes.

■ If you also have problems with the cervical vertebrae treat those relevant points too (see page 83).

Gall-bladder disorders

The gall-bladder is a small pouch attached to the liver which aids digestion. A poorly functioning gall-bladder can result in indigestion and flatulence. The gall-bladder can become inflamed and cause attacks of colic. In some cases small hard deposits known as gall-stones can form, which can be extremely painful. If you do have gallstones proceed with care: acupressure treatment could cause them to move about.

Treatment

▶ If you have a painful attack – possibly brought on by fatty food, or exertion and worry – try to relax before starting acupressure treatment and use steady but gentle pressure.

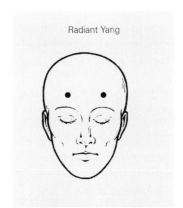

Radiant Yang

● Radiant Yang (one-and-a-half finger widths above the centre of the eyebrows). For colic, the left side is usually more successful than the right. Press – medium but constant pressure, until treatment has an effect, then press strongly, 5 minutes.

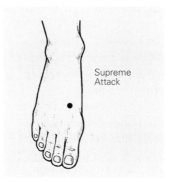

Supreme Attack

● Supreme Attack. For colic attacks. Press – strong pressure, 3-5 minutes.

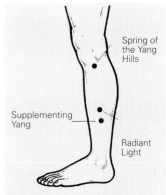

Spring of the Yang Hills

Supplementing Yang

Radiant Light

● Spring of the Yang Hills (= master point of the gall-bladder, slightly in front of the fibula head, that you can clearly feel). Press/merge, towards the ankle – strong pressure, 5 minutes.
● Radiant Light. Press/merge – strong pressure, 5 minutes.
● Supplementing Yang. Press/merge – strong pressure, up to 10 minutes.

Headaches, migraine, pains in the forehead

A headache is not an illness, it is a symptom. Headaches and migraine can have many causes – from tiredness to hunger, weather conditions to a slow gall-bladder function. They can however, especially in the case of women, be caused by hormones.

A headache tells the body that something is not in order – the pain is an alarm signal. This is why it is no use just treating a headache with medication. You also need to work out the cause.

There are four main types of headache:

● Sporadic headaches caused by a stressful situation (here all you usually need is quiet, relaxation and fresh air).

● Headaches caused by an organic disorder, such as a stomach complaint. A doctor must cure the cause.

● Migraine, which is a severe headache that returns periodically and is often accompanied by sensitivity to light, vision disorders and vomiting.

● Headaches that occur after an injury.

For treatment to work, the cause of the headache or migraine must be known. Then you can find out which pressure points are best for soothing the headache.

■ If you have constant or constantly recurring headaches you must consult your doctor.

When you get a headache you need to consider whether you are feeling stressed or if you are under any mental strain. We often overstrain our minds by keeping everything bottled up inside us, or by taking too much on.

Headaches are also a symptom of a disturbed balance between the area of understanding and feeling or between thinking and doing. You can get a headache if you are confused or frustrated. The head itself is hardly ever to blame for the pain, and orthodox medicine that relies on eliminating symptoms is not an effective means of curing the cause of pain. Nor can it help you with preventative measures. Painkilling medicines often have strong side-effects and only eliminate the symptoms for a short span of time. These medications should really only be taken as an emergency in exceptional circumstances.

■ Make sure you eat healthily and that you always give your food time to digest well. Take plenty of exercise in the fresh air and always try to balance bodily and mental exertion with relaxation.

Treatment

▶ Acupressure can help relieve pains on the top and at the back of the head (also see spinal cord problems page 83).

Please note:

Do not press more than one point at a time. When you have a headache wait about 20 minutes between each point.

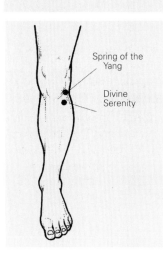

● Spring of the Yang. Soothes cramp. Press – strong pressure, 10 minutes.
● Divine Serenity. Press – strong pressure, 10 minutes.

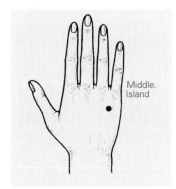

● Middle Island (two finger widths under ring finger). Press – medium pressure, 5 minutes.

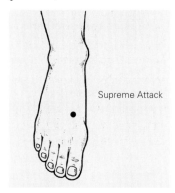

● Supreme Attack. For when the pain is strong. Press – strong pressure, as often as required.

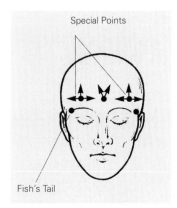

● Special Points. Eases the pain evenly in all directions. Press/rub, when required.
● Fish's Tail (slight bump at end of the eyebrow). Effective when you have a tension headache or a migraine. Press – medium pressure, 5 minutes.

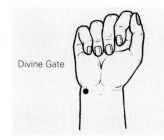

● Divine Gate (= balancing point of energy). Press – medium pressure, 5 minutes.

Headaches, migraine, pains in the forehead

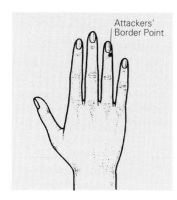

Attackers'
Border Point

● Attackers' Border Point.
Especially effective for
tension headaches. Press –
strong pressure, 3 times.

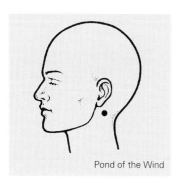

Pond of the Wind

● Pond of the Wind
(under the skull, between
the turning point of head
and the trapeze muscle).

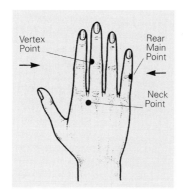

Vertex
Point

Rear
Main
Point

Neck
Point

Press – medium pressure, 3
minutes.
● Vertex Point
(inside middle finger, at the
middle joint) and Rear –
Main Point (outside little
finger at the middle joint).
Follow the direction of
arrow. Press – strong
pressure, 5 minutes.
● Neck Point
(right between the knuckles).
Press – strong pressure, 5
minutes.

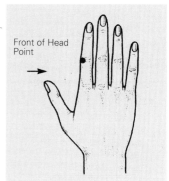

Front of Head
Point

● Front of Head Point (on
the inside of the index finger
at the middle joint). Follow
the direction of arrow. Press
– strong pressure,
5-10 minutes.

■ If you find that treating
these points is not
successful, you should go to
your doctor. Recurring or
constant headaches are often
due to organic disorders or
to a constant strain that can
lead to organic disorders.

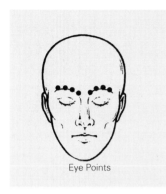

Eye Points

● Eye Points.
Effective against migraine.
Press every eye point from
inside to out separately; in
addition to this rub the
other points of pain carefully
– gentle pressure, when
required.

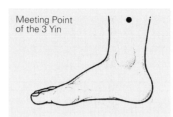

Meeting Point
of the 3 Yin

● Meeting Point of the 3 Yin.
Use when hormone
complaints cause a
headache, or when you have
a headache in connection
with menstruation.
Press/part – gentle pressure,
5-10 minutes.

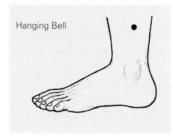

Hanging Bell

● Hanging Bell
(five finger widths over the
upper tip of the ankle at the
side of the fibula). Relieves
tension. Press – medium
pressure, 3 minutes.

■ Usually headaches are a
sign of stress. As every
person reacts differently to
stress it may take a while for
you find the points that
respond well to treatment.

For people who have a
headache due to nervous
tension or a feeling of
unease, treating the points
Divine Serenity or the
Divine Gate will be more
successful than for women
who have a headache mainly
due to the menstrual cycle.
In this case treating the
Meeting Point of the 3 Yin
will have the desired effect.

Take your time to discover
your special combination of
points.

Haemorrhoids

Haemorrhoids are swollen veins in the region of the rectum and anus. They cause irritation, pain and even bleeding, especially during and just after moving the bowels. Common causes of haemorrhoids include weakness of the vein tissue, and poor nourishment resulting in constipation or lack of bowel movement. Pregnant women also frequently suffer from haemorrhoids due to the internal pressure of the growing baby.

Treatment

▶ Acupressure treatment can alleviate the pain felt when sitting down or during a bowel movement, as well as the irritation and itch often suffered.

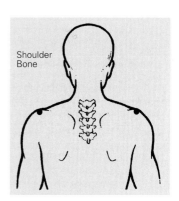

● Shoulder Bone
(in the divot above the shoulder joint).
Especially effective against itchiness; influences the vein system of the skin.
Press – strong pressure, 5-10 minutes.

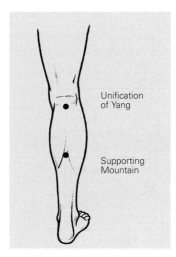

● Unification of Yang
(two finger widths beneath the central point at the back of the knee).
Press/merge, towards heel – medium pressure, 3 minutes.
● Supporting Mountain
(in the centre of the rise in the twin muscle). Treat simultaneously on both legs with the thumbs.
Press/merge – strong pressure, up to 10 minutes.

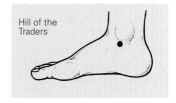

● Hill of the Traders.
For general strengthening of the connective tissue.
Press – medium pressure, 5-10 minutes.

Insomnia

Insomnia is often the beginning of a vicious circle of changing waking and sleeping patterns. It is commonly a symptom of other problems, but can in turn be the cause of further disorders.

With acupressure, difficulty in falling asleep can be just as effectively treated as difficulties during sleep. The inability to fall asleep usually occurs because of excess brain activity or psychological strain.

■ Sleeping tablets seem to be the only answer to insomnia for many people. But it is much better to find a natural alternative to your sleep problem.

Treatment

▶ The aim of the acupressure is to recreate inner calmness through physical harmonisation. This means that the intake of sleeping drugs can be avoided (see also nervousness and anxiety attacks, pages 73 and 44).

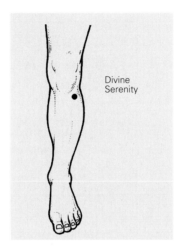

● Divine Serenity. Press slowly and with full concentration – strong pressure, 10 minutes.

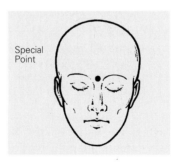

● Special Point (between the eyebrows). Press slowly and with full concentration – gentle pressure, 3-5 minutes.

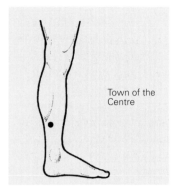

● Town of the Centre. Press/merge slowly and with full concentration– medium pressure, 5 minutes.

Please pay attention:

For difficulty in falling asleep, press Special Point and Divine Serenity. For difficulty in staying asleep, press Town of the Centre and Divine Serenity. (See also lack of concentration, page 92.)

Joint pain

Apart from physical injuries, such as sprains and breaks, the primary cause of joint pain is arthritis, which causes inflammation of the joints. The causes of arthritis are not entirely understood, but include general wear and tear of the body, physical predisposition, poor or inappropriate diet, or the delayed result of injury. It commonly occurs in the joints most under stress, such as hips, knees, spine and fingers. Unless the joints are acutely inflamed, exercise of the affected joints is vital. Acupressure can help to maintain movement.

Treatment

▶ Acupressure can help to treat pains in the joints resulting from inflammation or infection. It can help restore movement and ease swelling and stiffness.

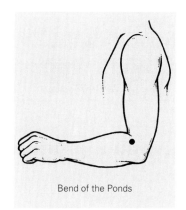

Bend of the Ponds

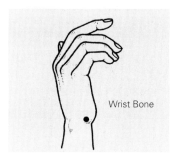

Wrist Bone

● Bend of the Ponds.
Press – medium pressure, up to 10 minutes.

● Wrist Bone.
Press – strong pressure, 5-10 minutes.

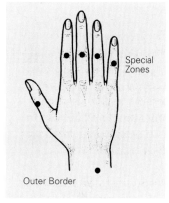

Special Zones

Outer Border

● Outer Border
(two finger widths behind the wrist, between the ulna and the radius).
Press – strong pressure, 5 minutes.
● Special Zones (directly on the finger joints).
Press with the thumb, strongly gripping the finger you are treating. If all the fingers on the hand are affected, the Chinese healing science stipulates treatment in the following order: ring finger, thumb, middle finger, index finger, little finger.
Press – medium pressure, 5-10 minutes.

Knee pain

The knee joint is frequently exposed to injuries and strain. Whether this is due to pains in the joints caused by old age and movement limitations, exertions at work, overexerting the knee joints during physical exercise, or through excess weight – acupressure cannot repair damage that already exists, but it does soothe pain considerably and can help to prevent further degeneration in individual cases. Lesser, irritating everyday complaints can often be eliminated. This can considerably improve the quality of life for older people. Short distances to the local shops and short walks or visits to friends can be done again without pain or discomfort.

■ Constant or frequent pain in the knees requires medical treatment and you should see your doctor.

Treatment

▶ The most important treatment is the "locus-do-lendi" therapy which is acupressure of the painful points.

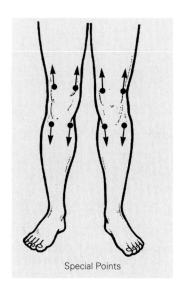

Special Points

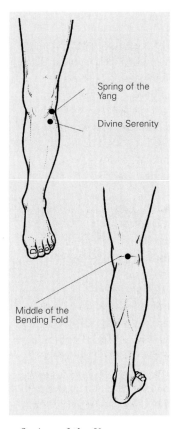

Spring of the Yang

Divine Serenity

Middle of the Bending Fold

● Special Points.
The four special points distribute and erase pain in the knee. Press/part – medium pressure, 5-15 minutes several times a day.

● Spring of the Yang (deep in front and under the head of the fibula). Press – strong pressure, 10 minutes.
● Divine Serenity.
Press – strong pressure, 5-15 minutes.
● Middle of the Bending Fold.
Press/part – medium pressure, 3 minutes.

Leg pain

Aching legs result from
strain of the muscles and
tendons, or from cramps
caused by a change in the
vascular system. If the pain
is accompanied by visible
swelling, it could also
indicate a disorder of the
heart or kidneys.

■ If in doubt, consult your
doctor so that vascular
changes or other functional
disorders can be treated
promptly.

It is your legs and feet that
carry you through life and
they symbolise the principle
of change and movement.
Sometimes foot or leg pain
can be a sign that some sort
of change is needed in your
life, or that something is
putting undue strain on you.

Treatment

▶ The pain of varicose
veins can be improved
through acupressure. In
ancient China, the Three
Mile Point was pressed by
soldiers during long foot
marches to relieve tiredness
and increase performance.

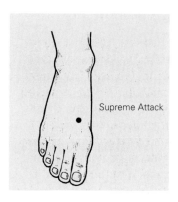

● Supreme Attack
(in the angle of the first and
second middle bones of the
foot). For swellings:
Push – medium pressure,
3-5 minutes.

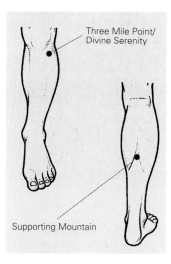

Three Mile Point/
Divine Serenity

Supporting Mountain

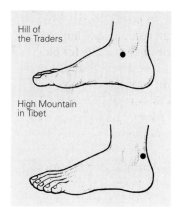

Hill of
the Traders

High Mountain
in Tibet

● Three Mile Point/Divine
Serenity. For cramps,
combine with Supporting
Mountain.
Press, in pairs, with a gentle
circular motion – medium
pressure, 10-15 minutes.
● Supporting Mountain
Press/part – strong pressure,
10 minutes.

● Hill of the Traders.
Press – medium pressure,
5 minutes.
● High Mountain in Tibet
(= master point of pain).
Press – medium pressure, up
to 10 minutes.

Menopause complaints

The body and the psyche have to adjust themselves to a changing hormone situation during the menopause. Signs of these hormonal changes are inner anxiety, hot flushes, frailty, and lack of energy. At sometime between the ages of 47 and 53 the ovaries stop functioning. If the hormones then fall below a certain level, you may need the help of medication, after a gynaecological examination, to re-establish a stable condition.

Please note:

Apart from being used as a preventative treatment, acupressure should always be applied when a side effect is noticeable.

Treatment

▶ The changing and adjusting processes of the body and the psyche during the menopause are supported by acupressing those points that have a harmonising and a stabilising effect. (See also Nervousness, page 73).

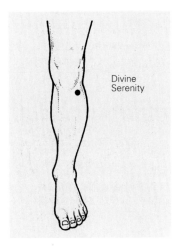

● Divine Serenity.
Press – medium pressure, 5-10 minutes.

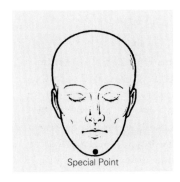

Special Point

● Special Point
(directly in the groove of the chin). Press – medium pressure, 3-5 minutes.

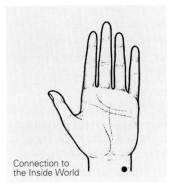

Connection to the Inside World

● Connection to the Inside World
(a width of a thumb underneath the wrist along the line of the little finger). Press – medium pressure, 3-5 minutes.

Menstruation complaints

Young women frequently suffer from irregular periods or period pains – often both together. These are usually caused by hormonal upsets. Psychical factors also have a lot to do with this. Pre-menstrual syndrome which includes complaints such as headaches, stomach-aches, backaches, swelling, rashes, depression, lethargy, irritability, weakening of the libido and even being more prone to accidents, can be particularly upsetting.

Treatment

▶ Acupressure harmonises your whole condition by activating the body's own control of hormone production (Hypothesise) which stabilises the hormone supply.

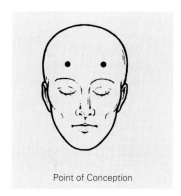

Point of Conception

● Point of Conception (three finger widths above the eyebrow line). Press – medium pressure, 5 minutes.

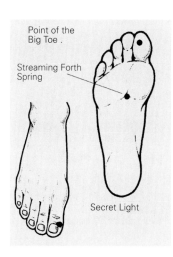

Point of the Big Toe .

Streaming Forth Spring

Secret Light

● Point of the Big Toe. Reflects the Hypothesise (brain gland, harmonic centre of direction). Press – medium pressure, 5-10 minutes.

● Streaming Forth Spring. Constant light pressure with the thumb soothes and relaxes. Get your partner to help. Press – gentle pressure, 10-15 minutes.
● Secret Light.
Use when bleeding is very heavy. Press – medium to strong pressure, 5 minutes.

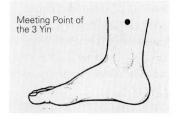

Meeting Point of the 3 Yin

● Meeting Point of the 3 Yin. Use when you get cramp during your period and when you have unspecified period pains. Press – begin with gentle pressure, 5-10 minutes.

Rest for 30 minutes after treating these points

Nasal cavity infection

The mucous membranes in the cavities (jaw, forehead and nostrils) are often chronically irritated. The slightest thing, like a draught or changes in temperature, can cause the infection to be severe (sinusitis). High sensitivity to pressure in the nasal cavity area, a blocked nose, a hoarse voice, headaches or high body temperature are side-effects. If the nasal cold lasts longer than a week, this usually points to a nasal cavity infection.

■ Your doctor should diagnose and treat a nasal cavity infection.

Acupressure eases a nasal cavity infection immediately and can, if applied in time, prevent the infection from spreading from the nose to the jaw and forehead.

A severe nasal cavity infection with side-effects can last up to three weeks, so treatment should begin when you feel the first signs.

Treatment

▶ Acupressure supports treatment with steam inhaling, warmth and nose drops that reduce swelling; if you apply over long periods of time you will find that the mucous membrane infection is cured.

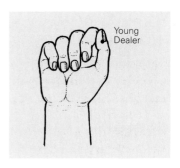

● Young Dealer.
Effective as a lymph point. Press – medium pressure, 3-5 minutes.

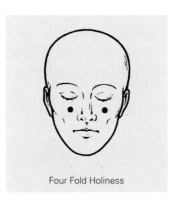

Four Fold Holiness

● Four Fold Holiness (you can feel them on a small bump). Press – gentle constant pressure, 3-5 minutes, up to 5 treatments a day.

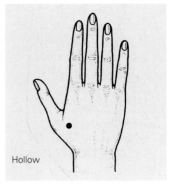

Hollow

● Hollow.
When the mucous membranes are irritated this has a healing effect. Press – medium to strong pressure, 5 minutes.

Nervousness, exhaustion

Nervous exhaustion – this diagnosis can be made fairly quickly. It means that due to a nervous condition you very quickly become exhausted or tired. It has several symptoms : excessive sweating, insomnia, anxiety without any cause or a general feeling of unease and fear. If disorders of the nervous system – regardless of what form – are in an advanced stage this is a clear sign that the body's own self-defence system cannot cope with some influence.

Treatment

▶ Acupressure regulates and harmonises the energies in the psycho-vegetative areas.

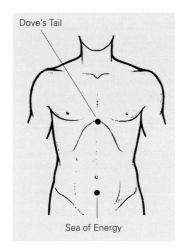

Dove's Tail

Sea of Energy

● Dove's Tail
(at the bottom end of the sternum). Press – medium pressure, 5-10 minutes.
● Sea of Energy.
Sets energy free, even when generally weak. Press – gentle to medium pressure, 5-10 minutes.

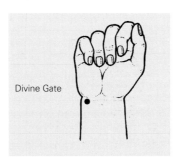

Divine Gate

● Divine Gate.
Press – medium pressure, 3-5 minutes.

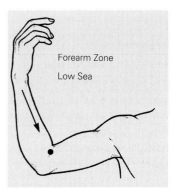

Forearm Zone

Low Sea

● Forearm Zone.
Push – towards elbow, 10 times per arm.
● Low Sea
(in the middle between the joint of the upper arm and the end of the elbow).
Press – 5 minutes.
● Divine Serenity
(see page 45). In the morning use blackcurrant herb oil (signal for activity), in the evening thistle oil (signal for peace).

Nicotine dependence

Smoking enhances the risk for many illnesses enormously. The risk of arteriosclerosis and a heart attack increases considerably, as do lung problems. Many smokers have a cough that is connected to this.

Acupressure helps to build up the nervous system. If you are strong enough to free yourself from nicotine dependency, smoking will be unnecessary as a balance to a lack of energy. However, smoking is often just a habit. In this case you should re-educate yourself and rather than pick up a cigarette turn to something else (for example acupressure).

The acupuncture of certain points of the ear is also noticeably successful. If you have ear acupuncture to fight nicotine dependence, make sure this is done by a qualified expert. The points on the ear have to be stuck to very precisely if the treatment is to be successful in the long term.

Treatment

▶ When you are trying to free yourself from a dependency many unpleasant withdrawal symptoms can be softened by applying acupressure.

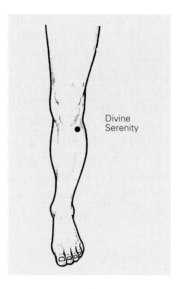

● Divine Serenity.
For balance and harmony.
Press – strong pressure,
10 minutes.

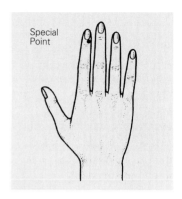

● Special Point
(to the bottom right of the fingernail on the index finger). Use when you feel your nerves are degenerating. Press – strong pressure, 5-10 minutes.

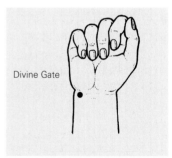

● Divine Gate.
Press – medium pressure,
5 minutes.

Nosebleeds

Nosebleeds are usually caused by something external such as a blow, fall, scratch or nose blowing; it is hardly ever the sign of a severe disorder. The most common cause is the dried up mucous membrane in the nose being burst. Should bleeding only occur from one nostril, the cause is usually in the nose itself, whilst bleeding from both nostrils may be due to a general disorder.

Treatment

▶ Generally nose bleeds stop after a few minutes of treatment. If the nosebleed continues and the blood loss is heavy, call your doctor.

General hints: Sit upright, do not talk, do not blow your nose, breathe slowly through your mouth, do not hold your head back. Place a bag of ice or a cloth soaked in cold water on the back of your neck, gently press the nostrils together.

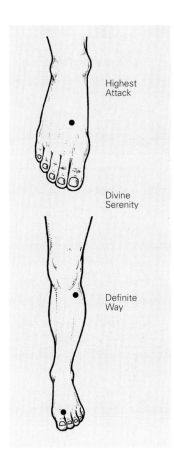

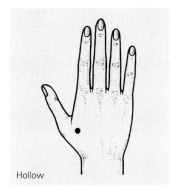

● Hollow
(= mucous membrane point). Most suitable for self-treatment. Press – strong pressure, 5 minutes.

Please note:

You must consult your doctor if:
● the nosebleed is heavy and will not stop
● the nosebleed is due to an injury to the head.

● Highest Attack and Divine Serenity.
Get your partner to apply these at the same time. Press – medium pressure, 5 minutes.
● Definite Way.
Press – strong pressure, 5 minutes.

Overweight

Eating behaviour is in most cases a mirror image of your psychological well-being. A voracious appetite, which can torment the overweight, is often nothing else but the longing for attention and affection, tenderness and security. This often starts with feeding as a baby – obesity often originates from educational patterns in early childhood towards eating behaviour. In only one to two per cent of cases is obesity caused through hormonal disorders. Being overweight is one of the main causes of heart attacks, diabetes, strokes, vascular disease and indigestion.

Treatment

▶ With acupressure you can activate important control centres for the appetite (see also vegetative malfunctioning, page 91).

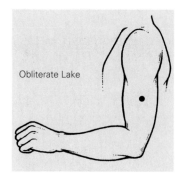

Obliterate Lake

● Obliterate Lake.
Press – gentle pressure,
30 seconds.

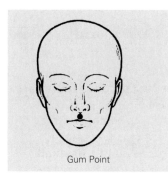

Gum Point

● Gum Point
(between upper lip and nostrils). Press – gentle pressure, 90 seconds.

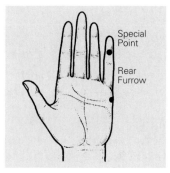

Special Point

Rear Furrow

● Special Point
(at the first joint of the little finger). Press in the rhythm of pulse acupress with the thumbnail – strong pressure, maximum of 20 seconds.
● Rear Furrow.
Press – strong pressure,
5 minutes.

A four week programme
● Rear Furrow and Defrosting Stream (page 56) should only be treated in the mornings (invigorating points).
● Gum Point and Obliterate Lake, should be acupressed gently for 30 seconds to prevent hunger.
● Divine Serenity (page 45) should also be acupressed.

Pain as a symptom

Doctors have only recently considered pain to be a valid symptom. Before this, pain was seen as the signal of a malfunction somewhere in the body (mechanistic pain theory), and pains outside the affected area were put down to misdirection in the nervous system. Successes of the needle-stitch analgesia and the discovery of the body's own painkillers, (endorphine) destroyed this theory. It is now known that pain is not necessarily caused by physical disorders and that the intensity of the pain does not necessarily depend on the seriousness of the injury.

Treatment

▶ Acupressure invigorates the production of the body's own painkiller.

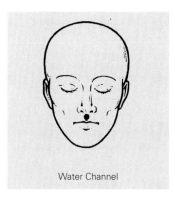

Water Channel

● Water Channel.
Particularly effective in treating acute pain.
Press – medium pressure, 3 minutes. Can also be acupressed in a 10 minute rhythm with the fingertip.

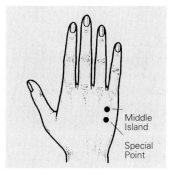

Middle Island

Special Point

● Middle Island.
Press – strong pressure, 5 minutes.
● Special Point.
Press – strong pressure, 2-5 minutes.

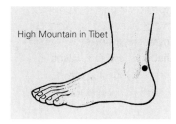

High Mountain in Tibet

● High Mountain in Tibet.
Treats a* * kinds of pain (main point). Press – medium to strong pressure, 5-10 minutes.
● Divine Serenity and Va* * ey Bottom (page 53). Press combined.

Prostate complaints

The prostate gland at the exit of the bladder surrounds the urethra and is about the size of a chestnut. Expansion and inflammation of this gland are the most common complaints. A prostate expansion constricts the bladder exit. Frequent urges to pass water, stinging when passing water, delayed start when trying to pass water, urinary dribbling, through to an inability to empty the bladder can all result from prostate problems.

Backache, frequent urges to pass water and difficulties with passing water, are symptoms of a prostate inflammation; it can easily become chronic. Prostate problems can also affect the psychological well-being by leading to nervousness and insomnia.

As soon as any of these symptoms occur you should consult your doctor. For any treatment to be successful, it is vital for the acute inflammation not to become chronic.

Treatment

▶ Acupressure can prevent prostate expansion or prostate inflammation from becoming chronic.

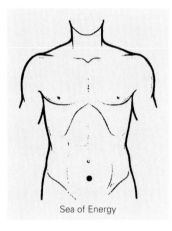

Sea of Energy

● Sea of energy.
This can also be effective through parting and combining. Press/part/merge – medium to strong pressure, up to 10 minutes.

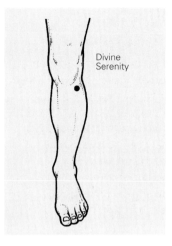

Divine Serenity

● Divine Serenity.
Press – medium pressure, 10 minutes.

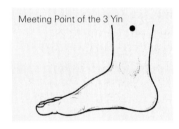

Meeting Point of the 3 Yin

● Meeting Point of the 3 Yin.
This has a harmonising effect onto the whole genital area. Press/part – medium pressure, 5 minutes.

Rheumatic complaints

Rheumatism is a common disease; extreme frequency and a great variety of original causes and the form it takes, as much as the fact that there is no effective orthodox medical rheumatism therapy, makes this illness a widespread health problem.

Limitation of movement, strong pains and swelling are just some of the complaints from which people with rheumatism suffer. The inflamed joint swelling is particularly painful; the most likely to be affected first are finger and toe joints. Wrists, knees and shoulders are often the next areas to become inflamed, if something is not done to prevent it.

■ If your doctor diagnoses rheumatism, acupressure can then be a valuable support to any treatment that he prescribes.

Treatment

▶ Acupressure affects the metabolism and helps to soothe pain (see also leg pains, page 69; joint pains, page 67; pain, page 77).

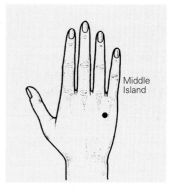

● Middle Island.
For fast pain relief and relief of tension. Press – if necessary.

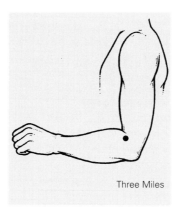

Three Miles

● Three Miles.
Will help relieve limitation of movement, pain or signs of paralysis. Press – medium pressure, 5 minutes.

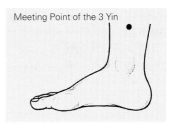

Meeting Point of the 3 Yin

● Meeting Point of the 3 Yin.
Press/part – medium pressure, 5 minutes.

Sciatica problems, lumbago

The sciatic nerve is one of the longest nerve cords in the human body; it runs from the area around the sacrum down to the toes. If a branch of the nerve is jammed (due to a slipped disc or a shift of the spine) the typical penetrating sciatica pain is accompanied by limited movement. If the nerve is trapped by the spinal cord, paralysis can occur. Sudden complaints that appear after an unfortunate movement of the body are referred to as "lumbago". The pain can become severe and should not be ignored (see spinal cord problems, page 83).

Treatment

▶ Acupressure soothes pain and loosens muscle tension.

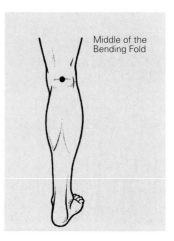

● Middle of the Bending Fold (in the middle of the back of the knee). Press/part – gentle to medium pressure, 3 minutes.

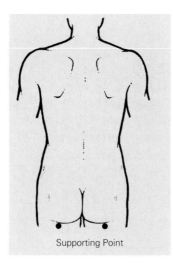

Supporting Point

● Supporting Point (acupressed by a partner whilst patient relaxes the stomach). Press/merge – strong pressure, up to 10 minutes.

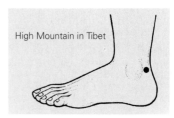

High Mountain in Tibet

● High Mountain in Tibet. Press in the direction of the heel when limbs hurt – strong pressure, 5 minutes.

Sexual disorders

Psychological problems, such as unconscious fears or difficulty with your partner, are the main causes of sexual disorders. This is why a purely medicinal therapy if often ineffective. A sexually fulfilled life is only possible if both partners are physically and emotionally relaxed and can live in an atmosphere which is free of fear, feelings of guilt or performance pressures. In women, the disorder is often hidden because a couple do not necessarily stop having intercourse (see also nervousness, page 73, anxiety attacks, page 44).

You should seek expert advice if these types of problems put a strain on either yourself or your relationship.

Treatment

▶ If it is possible for you and your partner to do the acupressure together, this could be the first step towards success.

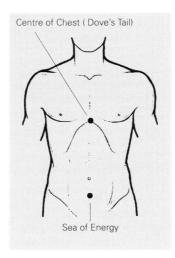

Centre of Chest (Dove's Tail)

Sea of Energy

● Centre of Chest (Dove's Tail).
For premature ejaculation this can be pressed before and during intercourse. Press – strong pressure, 5 minutes.
● Sea of Energy.
Press – medium pressure, 5 minutes.

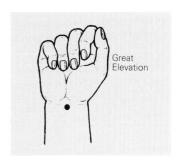

Great Elevation

● Great Elevation.
Takes care of the psychological balance (as well as Divine Serenity, page 45). Press – medium pressure, 5 minutes.

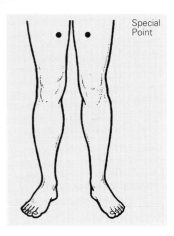

Special Point

● Special Point
(on the thighs). Suitable for frigidity and the inability to ejaculate. Press/part/merge – medium pressure, 5-10 minutes.

Sore throat

A sore throat can have many causes. It is most commonly a side-effect or symptom of another complaint, such as a cold infection or tonsillitis.

Both children and adults often suffer from an inflamed and sore throat. A "stabbing" sore throat with loss of appetite, problems swallowing and a dry feeling in the throat can signal the onset of an acute gum or tonsil infection; fever, swollen lymph glands at the lower jaw angle, and swelling of the tonsils may also occur. If the sore throat is the result of a cold, the sooner you apply acupressure the better, as it will help to ease the discomfort.

■ An acute or severe sore throat with feelings of choking or difficulty in swallowing should be looked at by a doctor.

Treatment

▶ Acupressure can help to soothe an uncomplicated sore throat, where the symptoms show hoarseness, slight problems with swallowing and are accompanied by a cold.

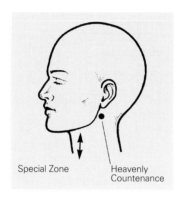

Special Zone   Heavenly
                      Countenance

● Special Zone.
Push – gentle pressure, 3-5 minutes.
● Heavenly Countenance.
Press – very gentle pressure, 1 minute.

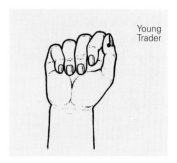

Young Trader

● Young Trader (= master point for the lung). Press with the thumbnail, several times a day – strong pressure, 5 minutes.

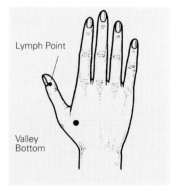

Lymph Point

Valley Bottom

● Lymph Point (on the thumb). Especially effective for the lymph system. Press – medium pressure, 5 minutes.
● Valley Bottom. Regulates the mucous membrane. Press – strong pressure, up to 10 minutes.

Spinal cord problems, shoulder and arm pain

The spinal cord is the most important axis for movement in the body. Disorders in the vicinity of the spinal cord limit movement within the whole human body. The range of disorders comprises everything from simple, tense muscles, that can be treated with massage, to problems with the discs and curvature of the spine.

■ Please consult your doctor if you have a back problem.

Good Training

Gently swing your spine round by bending and stretching in all directions, like a cat after it wakes up. This makes sure that all your discs fall into place properly (see also backpains, page 47; pains, page 77).

The treatment

▶ Complaints in the vicinity of your spinal column can definitely be soothed by applying acupressure.

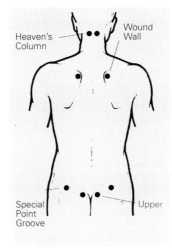

● Heaven's Column.
Press/part/merge – medium pressure, 5 minutes.
● Special Point.
Press – gentle to strong pressure, 10-15 minutes.
● Wound Wall
(at the inner upper end of the shoulder blade).
Press/part – medium pressure, 5 minutes.
● Upper Groove.
Press/part/merge – medium pressure, 5-10 minutes.

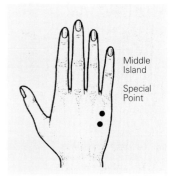

● Middle Island and Special Point.
Press – strong pressure, 5 minutes.

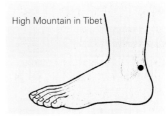

● High Mountain in Tibet.
Press – strong pressure, 5 minutes.

■ Rub all painful points and zones with gentle pressure. In addition acupress High Mountain of Tibet and Special Point on the back of the hand.

Stomach-aches

Unspecified stomach-aches can be caused either by disturbances in the digestive system or by psychological tension. In the former, the organs adjoining the digestive system are often affected. General indisposition, a feeling of being too full, stomach pain, flatulence and problems with bowel movement can occur.

■ If you have persistent stomach-aches over a period of time, consult your doctor to discover the exact cause of the problem.

The stomach meridian is closely connected with our emotional experience. Treatment of the harmonisation points for this meridian can be effective when emotional stresses are at the root of the digestive problems.

Treatment

▶ If the stomach-aches are caused by ulcers or infection, then acupressure cannot cure the problem, it can only soothe the pain. If, however, the stomach-aches are caused by muscular cramps or by inefficient gastric juices in the digestive process, acupressure can bring about lasting relief.

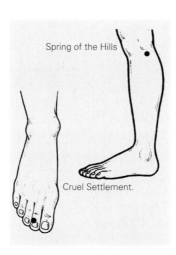

● Spring of the Hills, (at the back of the shin in a clear noticeable curve). Press/part – 5-10 minutes.
● Cruel Settlement (= harmonisation point for the stomach). Press – strong pressure, 5-10 minutes.

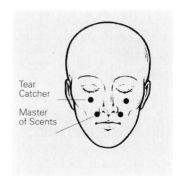

● Tear Catcher (= harmonisation point for the stomach). Press – gentle pressure, 5 minutes.
● Master of Scents (mucous membrane point, left and right of the nostrils). Press – starting gently, 5 minutes.

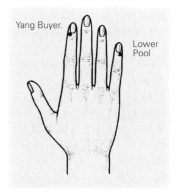

● Yang Buyer and Lower Pool (= harmonisation points for the bowel). Press – medium strength, 5-8 minutes.

Stomach intestine disorders

Infections of the mucous membranes are amongst the most common disorders in the process of digestion. Temporary everyday stomach complaints are usually due to irritations of the mucous membranes. Nervous impulses cause the stomach wall to produce too much acid and the mucous membranes become irritated and infected. Figures of speech such as: "that has gone right to my stomach" – "I'll need to digest that" – refer to the close connection between mental sensation and a bodily reaction.

Natural means of healing are generally more effective than orthodox treatments that only consist of chemically neutralising the excess stomach acid; though acid-binding medications do soothe pain, they disturb the process of digestion at the same time.

Natural therapies should be able to prevent the over-production of acid.

To make the movement of the bowels function normally a balanced diet, high in fibre is very important. You may find that a light diet helps to ease the digestion and soothe the pain, however it does not help cure the cause of the problem.

■ Your doctor should diagnose disorders of the stomach and intestine.

Treatment

▶ Slight stomach mucous-membrane infections can be cleared within 3 to 7 days using acupressure.

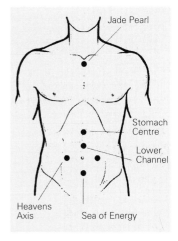

● Heavens Axis
(three finger widths from the navel). Press/part – medium pressure, 5 minutes.
● Jade Pearl and Stomach Centre.
Press together when burping (heartburn) – gentle pressure, 3 minutes.
● Stomach centre.
Press/part – medium pressure, 5 minutes.
● Lower Channel.
Good when you get cramps. Press/part – medium pressure, 5-10 minutes.
● Sea of Energy
(three finger widths from the navel). Press – medium to strong pressure, 3 minutes.

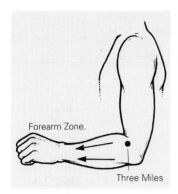

● Forearm Zone.
Push towards wrist,
7 minutes.
● Three Miles.
Press – medium to strong
pressure, 10 minutes.

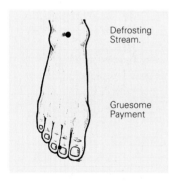

● Defrosting Stream.
Press – strong pressure,
5 minutes.
● Gruesome Payment
(= harmonising point). Get
your partner to do this when
you are in bed. Press – strong
pressure, 3-5 minutes.

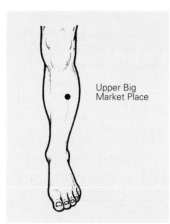

● Upper Big Market Place
(two finger widths above the
middle between ankle and
knee joint). Use when you
have wind and feel full.
Press/merge – medium
pressure, 10 minutes.

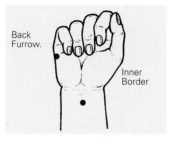

● Back Furrow
(on the outside of the inner
hand). Press – strong
pressure, 5 minutes.
● Inner Border
(three finger widths below
the wrist). Press – start with
gentle pressure, 3 minutes.

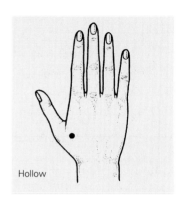

● Hollow
(below thumb and index
finger). Soothes the mucous
membranes and normalises
their functions. Press –
strong pressure, up to 10
minutes.
● Divine Serenity
(energy point with
harmonising effect, see page
45). Can be pressed in
addition to the other points.

Stutter

It is an interesting fact that about four times as many men stutter as women. This type of speech disorder is not genetically transmitted, even though stutters appear more often within one family. In most cases, there is a psychological reason for the stutter (see anxiety attacks, page 44).

Stuttering is caused, in most cases, through fear and nervous tensions.

With children it is a development and speech disorder, which should not be worsened by constantly correcting the child. (Family tensions and conflicts give a higher tendency for stuttering).

Should your child have a speech problem it is sensible to look for the original cause. Your doctor will be able to advise you on the best course of action.

Treatment

▶ Along with speech therapy, you work on the psychogeneric prerequisites with acupressure, in order to balance breathing and speech. Children should learn to treat themselves, as the long-term acupressure of all points every morning and evening promises to be very successful.

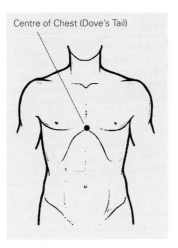
Centre of Chest (Dove's Tail)

● Centre of Chest (Dove's Tail).
Press – medium pressure, 10 minutes.

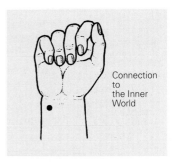
Connection to the Inner World

● Connection to the Inner World (one width of a thumb above the wrist). Press – medium pressure, up to 5 minutes.

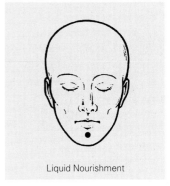
Liquid Nourishment

● Liquid Nourishment (between lower lip and the end of the chin). Press – strong pressure, 2-3 minutes. Additionally, acupress the point Divine Serenity (see page 45).

Tiredness

Tiredness and lack of energy are usually side-effects of other disorders or symptoms of, for example, circulation problems, flu infections, problems with digestion or feeling tense.

■ Constant tiredness and lack of motivation can also be due to a poor diet or a malfunctioning thyroid gland or liver. Seek advice from your doctor if you suffer from persistent tiredness.

Tiredness can also be a bodily reaction to your everyday life. If you are too busy and stressed you are likely to be lacking in energy and will find it hard to relax. Acupressure can help relieve stress and replenish your energy levels.

Treatment

▶ Acupressure stimulates the circulation and temporarily frees energy reserves – do not under any circumstances be wasteful with these reserves. Make sure you get enough peace and quiet, relaxation and sleep.

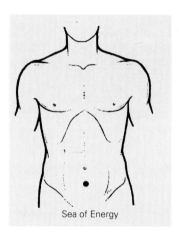
Sea of Energy

● Sea of Energy.
Pinch – medium pressure, 5-10 minutes.

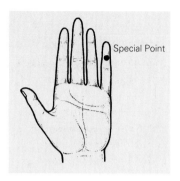
Special Point

● Special Point
(at the first joint of the little finger). Press with the thumbnail as required – strong pressure, maximum of 30 seconds.

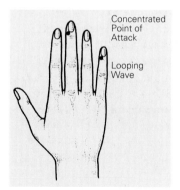
Concentrated Point of Attack

Looping Wave

● Concentrated Point of Attack and Looping Wave. Press – strong pressure, 5 minutes.
● Acupress Divine Serenity and Three Miles (page 45 and 79) in addition to the above points.

Toothache

Apart from a headache, toothache is probably the most common pain there is.

Naturally, acupressure does not replace any treatment a dentist could give. However, if the pain suddenly erupts or starts during the week-end, you can soothe it with acupressure. Acupressure is also very useful (especially at night) if you have to spend a long time waiting for treatment.

More recent methods of analysis have shown that some toothache has little to do with the teeth themselves, but is caused by diseased organs. Therefore, if there is no damage to any tooth, toothache may be an indication of a disease or illness.

Treatment

▶ By stimulating two points (Gum Point in the mouth and Yang Buyer on the index finger) the passage of the pain is briefly interrupted and the production of the body's own pain killer is stimulated.

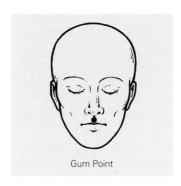

Gum Point

● Gum Point.
This can be acupressed from both the outside (press on the upper lip) and also the inside (press directly on the gum). Press – gentle to medium pressure, 2-5 minutes.

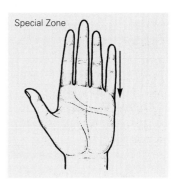

Special Zone

● Special Zone
(on the outside of the little finger). Good for children. Push – 5-7 minutes.

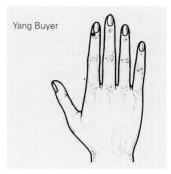

Yang Buyer

● Yang Buyer
(at the bottom of the nail of the index finger). Good for soothing pain when you are being treated by your dentist. Press using thumbnail – strong pressure, as required.

Travel sickness
Seasickness

Strong perspiration, nausea, vomiting or circulation trouble are side-effects of this disorder. The cause is a misdirection of the meteoric impulses of the nerves.

Intensive focusing on a particular point of reference usually helps to fight the nausea (with an upset stomach, never suppress the vomiting).

Frequent vomiting leads to a loss of body fluids and minerals, which can be highly dangerous if not compensated immediately with unsweetened herbal tea with added salt, or a rehydration solution from the pharmacy.

Treatment

▶ Acupressure has a calming effect on the mechanical activity of the digestive system and gives you a more relaxed and calm attitude towards the way you are feeling.

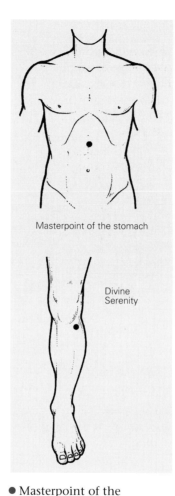

Masterpoint of the stomach

Divine Serenity

● Masterpoint of the Stomach and Divine Serenity.
Press – begin with gentle pressure and then gradually build up to strong pressure, 5-10 minutes.

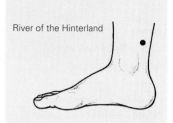

River of the Hinterland

● River of the Hinterland (two finger widths wide above the point of the inner ankle, next to the Achilles tendon).
Press – strong pressure, 5 minutes.

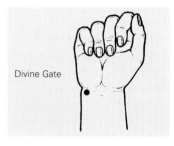

Divine Gate

● Divine Gate
(= balancing point of energy). Press – medium pressure,
5 minutes.

Vegetative disorders, vegetative dystonia

These are all the unconscious malfunctions of the vegetative nervous system – regardless of what kind of bodily symptoms they express themselves as.

In orthodox medicine vegetative dystonia is diagnosed when general disorders such as headaches, insomnia, circulation problems or dizziness occur without any specific organic disorder being found. At first the complaints are harmless, but they can, if they are not treated by a doctor, lead to lasting disorders of the nervous system. The reason for many types of vegetative disorders is an uneven balance between tension and relaxation.

Try to avoid anything that puts you under pressure in the first instance, and consciously look for ways to relax, so that you are calmer and therefore feel more stable again.

Treatment

▶ Acupressure helps you to have a more relaxed approach to everyday problems which in turn helps to boost your self-confidence.

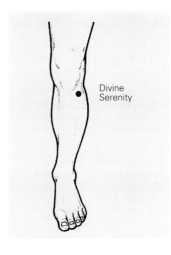

Divine Serenity.
Press – medium pressure, 10 minutes.

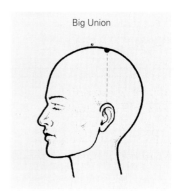

Big Union

● Big Union.
Press – gentle pressure, 3-5 minutes.

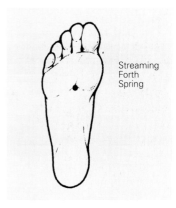

Streaming Forth Spring

● Streaming Forth Spring.
Acupress whilst in a relaxed position, by a partner with the ball of their thumb. Press – gentle pressure, 2 minutes.

Weakness in concentration

There are many outside distractions which can affect us during the course of a day, making it difficult for us to concentrate on what we are supposed to be doing. This lack of concentration can be a problem, especially if we are studying, or doing detailed work.

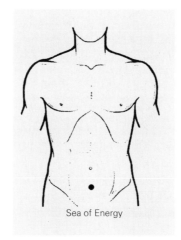

Sea of Energy

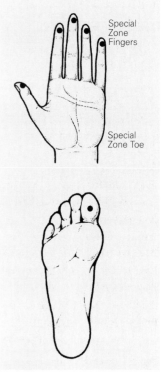

Special Zone Fingers

Special Zone Toe

Treatment

▶ If the lack of concentration is not due to a malfunction in the brain that only the doctor can diagnose or treat, acupressure will help to balance deficits of energy in the mind.

Schoolchildren with concentration disorders can benefit from having acupressure quietly every morning for 10 minutes before setting off for school.

● Sea of Energy (= main point of energy two to three finger widths underneath the navel).
Press/partition by pinching with the thumb and index finger – gentle to medium pressure, 5 minutes.

● Special Zone Fingers and Special Zone Toe.
Press in the morning and in the evening – medium pressure, 5 to 10 minutes.

■ Both points have a reflexive relationship to the hypothesise, that is the directing centre of all hormonal glands.

Complaints and Subject Index

Published originally under the title "Akupressur" by Gräfe und Unzer Verlag GmbH, Munich
© 1994 Dr Sigrid Flade, D-83700 Rottach-Weissach

Authorized English language edition published by
Time-Life Books BV, 1066 Amsterdam
© 1997 Time-Life Books BV
First English language printing 1997

English translation by Carmona UK
Editorial Manager: Christine Noble
Editor: Alison Mackonochie
Layout/DTP: Dawn McGinn

ISBN 0 7054 3521 0

20 19 18 17 16 15 14 13 12 11 10 9 8 7 6 5 4 3 2 1